LOVE &

ROSES

from

DAVID

LOVE &
ROSES
from
DAVID

A LEGACY OF LIVING AND DYING

BY ROBERT J. GRANT

A.R.E. Press   •   Virginia Beach   •   Virginia

A.R.E. Press
Sixty-Eighth & Atlantic Avenue
P.O. Box 656
Virginia Beach, VA 23451-0656

Grateful acknowledgment is made to the following publishers for permission to reprint from their publications:

On Death and Dying, copyright 1969 by Elisabeth Kübler-Ross. Macmillan Publishing Company. Used by permission.
And the Band Played On: Politics, People, and the AIDS Epidemic by Randy Shilts, copyright 1987, St. Martin's Press. Used by permission.
Reflections on Life After Life by Raymond A. Moody, Jr., M.D., copyright 1977, Mockingbird/Bantam Books. Used by permission.

Edgar Cayce Readings © 1971, 1993 by the Edgar Cayce Foundation.
All rights reserved.

Library of Congress Cataloging-in-Publication Data
Grant, Robert J.
    Love and roses from David: a legacy of living and dying/by Robert J. Grant.
        p.   cm.
    Includes bibliographical references.
    ISBN 0-87604-311-2
    1. AIDS (Disease). 2. Terminal care. I. Title.
RC607.A26G63   1994
362.1'969792-dc20   93-28528

Cover design by Patti McCambridge
Cover illustration by Lisa Agnes Windham

For Mary-Margaret Hicks

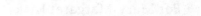

For . . . it is not all of life to live, nor yet all of death to die. For life and death are one, and only those who will consider the experience as one may come to understand or comprehend what peace indeed means.

Edgar Cayce
August 18, 1939

Acknowledgments

There are many people who have been guiding lights for me during the development and birth of this book. Special thanks to my longtime friends and mentors, Lois I. Bennett and Darrell L. Cook, both of whom gave me love, strength, and encouragement through my darkest hours. Warm gratitude to two psychologists who are far ahead of their time, G. Scott Sparrow and Henry Reed; their friendship, counseling, and insights have been invaluable to me. Very special thanks to Dr. Elisabeth Kübler-Ross, who inspired my work with the terminally ill. Loving thanks to my father and mother, George and Mary Lou Grant, who gave me my independence, my wings to fly. I would like to especially thank Joseph Dunn, my patient editor and friend, who motivated and inspired me to write this book. A special note of thanks to all my friends with AIDS who shared with me the story of their lives in the midst of their dying—a selfless, priceless gift. I love and miss you all.

Author's Note

*T*he time I spent with David—the last six months of his life—represents a culmination of unusual experiences that led to a glimpse of the nature of life and the mystery of death and the processes of dying. The backdrop of this book is a chronicle of those experiences before I met David and became an intimate part of his family.

The dialogues in *Love and Roses from David* have been taken with permission from my personal journals, interviews, and recorded conversations. For purposes of narrative flow, I have reconstructed dialogue and conversations from the above sources and, of course, my memory. The content of the dialogues and the characters are factual. In order to protect confidentiality, however, certain names and places have been changed or their characteristics altered. Only first names are used in the dialogues of the AIDS support group meetings.

Portions of this book have been previously published in *Venture Inward* magazine, July/August 1990, and are used by permission.

Robert J. Grant
December 1993

1

◆

*F*ear. It was born early in my preadolescent years. It lived a fruitful life well into my adulthood. But the instilled fear taught me a great deal and forced me to search for answers. Not an enjoyable journey at times, but a necessary one. Above all else, it was never dull.

My quest to understand the nature of death, dying, survival of the soul—the universal questions—was not a search for which I volunteered. Rather it began with a Baptist minister whose living depended upon the salvation of "God's children." This minister went to dramatic lengths to be about his business of salvation. A tool he used to reach that end was fear.

Now, some twenty years since my first encounter with the clergy, I can recall that meeting with a clarity and a certain amount of cynical humor. But then, I was a twelve-

year-old kid, and that clergyman scared the hell out of me.
From my present age of thirty-two, this is how I remember
it:

A minister pulled up alongside the twelve-year-old
blond boy who was riding his bicycle along Lake Ever-
green in rural Indiana. The minister was driving a
battered Dodge four-door that had seen better days.
Although the boy did not go to church, he knew the
older gentleman was a minister—he wore a gold cru-
cifix around his neck. Bibles were lying haphazard in
the passenger seat and in the back seat. The reverend
had a weathered face and wore a wrinkled suit. He had
a kindly smile.
   "Son, I've got some good news for you," he said,
smiling. He got out of his car and stretched.
   "What's that?" the boy asked.
   "I'm here on the Lord's work," the minister replied,
handing the boy one of the pocket-sized Bibles.
"Spreading the word of Jesus' salvation." The boy was
not uneasy. He had seen these traveling ministers stop
off at friends' houses. Very active Baptists, they usually
traveled on foot, Bibles in hand. He was going to make
the boy late. Supper was always at 5:30 p.m. The sun
was slowly descending over the trees on Lake Ever-
green. Whatever "good news" he was going to give, he
needed to hurry it up.
   "Have you got time, son?" he asked.
   "Not much. If I'm late, I'll get in trouble."
   The minister wasn't bothered one bit by this. A smile
spread across his sun-worn face. "Then I'll get to the
point. Let me read you something." He opened his
Bible, a larger version of the pocket-sized models he
had in the car. The book opened at a marked spot, re-
vealing a large picture of Jesus on the cross. The details

of the picture shocked the boy. Christ's tortured eyes turned to the sky, blood poured from His downturned mouth, and He appeared to be screaming. Usually, the boy liked seeing pictures of Jesus—especially the one of Him carrying the lost lamb. When the boy would visit his grandmother's home, he would always run into her den to look at the pictures in her little Bible. She kept it on the secretary, and he would gaze at the drawings of Jesus. The pictures made him feel happy inside; this picture made him feel awful.

"But if we walk in the light," the minister read aloud, "as he is in the light, we have fellowship one with another, and the blood of Jesus Christ his Son cleanseth us from all sin.

"If we say that we have no sin, we deceive ourselves, and the truth is not in us. If we confess our sins, he is faithful and just to forgive us our sins, and to cleanse us from all unrighteousness. If we say that we have not sinned, we make him a liar, and his word is not in us." (I John 1:7-9)

He leveled his eyes at the boy.

"Do you make Jesus a liar?"

"What? No! I'm no liar. What are you—?" The boy was alarmed and angry. He backed up a step, holding tightly to the handlebars of his bike. Seeing the boy's unease, the minister replaced his sternness with a smile.

"Of course, you're not. Only people who say they're not sinners make Him a liar." The boy was trying to digest what the minister was saying—but it made little sense; he only felt confused and hurt.

"All you have to do is confess that Jesus is the Savior, that you accept Him into your heart, and confess you're a sinner. You'll be spared the agony of eternal hellfire when you leave this world." The minister again looked at the boy solemnly. His gaze was hypnotic. His expressions changed with lightning speed; when he wasn't smiling, he didn't look pleasant at all. Smiling, he looked like a kindly old man. The boy was transfixed.

The boy accepted that the minister was indeed on "the Lord's work." Yet he felt fearful, and a sense of dread overcame him while looking into the minister's eyes. The boy did not want to look and yet he couldn't not look; similar to a deer who is frozen, hypnotized by the headlights of an oncoming car. The boy was too scared to speak—but too intrigued to run.

"Do you know what hell is like?" the minister asked.

"No," the boy whispered. His eyes kept returning to the picture of Christ in agony. It looked alive and sinister. He had never seen such a graphic portrayal of the Crucifixion. Christ looked haunted, tortured, and betrayed in this picture. It was a depiction that would haunt the boy's dreams for years.

"Why, hell is a thousand times worse than that picture. You never rest. You burn forever. Most people are going to burn. They're going to burn because they're not saved." He placed his hand on the boy's shoulder and looked at him gravely.

"Jesus looks like that in this picture," he said in his low, minister's voice, "because He's taken on all the agonies of hell for you. It's all been done. He died for you. But you have to confess your sins, realize you are a sinner, and accept Christ into your heart—or else . . . " His words trailed off, and the boy looked back to the agonized Christ.

Or else? The boy had never heard any of this during his religious education classes in school—and his mother's Bible stories never ended with "or else." The boy was rooted to the spot beside the minister, the minister who had been sent by God to help the boy.

The minister elaborated about sin; he talked of "lust, greed, deception"—words that had a foreign sound to the boy's ears. The words were lost on the boy—he didn't know anything except that sin was the bad things that bad people did. He tried to conjure up his "sins." The boy had lied to his parents a couple of times. He didn't like his teacher at school. He had looked at several *Playboy* magazines. He got mad and fought with his brothers. After mulling these things over, the boy looked up at the minister.

"What do I do?" the boy asked.

"Repeat these words."

It seemed eerie that the boy and the minister were alone. There, while thinking of the picture of the crucified Christ, the boy prayed. He repeated the words the minister said, accepting Christ into his heart, and admitted to being a sinner, asked for forgiveness of his "sins," even though the boy had just got acquainted with them.

The minister put his hands on the boy's head and began praying loudly. The boy hoped no one was nearby. Part of him was frightened. Part of him felt ridiculous.

"Hear the prayer of Your servant!" the minister crowed. "Save him from the fires of eternal hell! Keep him always, Lord. Let him not falter! Amen!" The boy was shaking.

The boy thought of his parents—wondering what they would think about all of this. His mom and dad didn't have much use for these ministers. But his folks were good people, and he told the minister just that, even though they weren't "saved." They would tell the boy Bible stories about Jesus. They told him the good stories, the ones about Jesus' miracles and the Golden

Rule. They never told him anything about salvation or hell or sinners. He wondered why.

"Doesn't matter how good people are," the minister said. "If they don't confess Jesus to be the Savior of the world, God will cast them into hell forever. He's patient and kind—but He loses His patience with people after a while."

This was a side of God the boy didn't know. He had heard God was eternally patient and kind. This business of hell frightened him. He was anxious. Burning forever, sin. The dark words rang in the boy's mind.

The minister was still rattling on about the wages of sin when the boy interrupted him. "I'm late, mister. Thanks a lot for . . . for everything."

"Here's a Bible for you. And take some of these Bible tracts," the minister said. "Be sure to read them—especially when you feel like you're backsliding. You're saved now; but you can always backslide. Don't go back to your old ways." He said this last sentence, pointing at the boy accusingly. What old ways? Backsliding?

"Give some of those tracts to your family and friends. Time is short! The Lord won't be patient for much longer!"

The boy got on his bicycle and rode toward home. He waved to the minister, who returned the boy's wave but did not smile. Riding homeward, the boy knew what being afraid was. Images of the crucified Christ—His tortured face looking heavenward—entered the boy's mind unbidden. He tried to think of eternity—forever—unending. He promised himself never to do anything wrong again—no fighting with his brothers, never lying to his parents, no dirty magazines. New emotions were awakened: fear, worry, anxiety. His young mind didn't have words for these emotions, but the feelings etched themselves deep in his psyche. Little did he know those fears would be harbored for many years. The boy's wondering mind was blossoming into a worrying one—preoccupied with the possibility of his eternal torment in hell. He silently prayed a child's prayer to a God he had never known—to spare him from such punishment.

———

The child was I. The fear was mine. My overactive imagination drew me again and again to the memories of the roadside minister; the face of Christ in pain; the sinister sound of the words *sin, hell, eternity.* Looking back, I realize how impressionable and sensitive I was. The minister's words became living things to my vivid imagination.

Most kids experience a fear of the dark. My remembrance of the darkness in those days was malevolent and full of frightening possibilities. As I look back, I can see that it was not the fear of hell or damnation that was awakened in me, but the fear of death itself. I began to fear the unknown and the unseen: death.

2

◆

*A*fter my experience with the minister, I was prone to
episodes of nightmares, night terrors, and sleep-
walking. Even now, as an adult, during stressful
times I occasionally walk in my sleep and awaken disori-
ented and confused. As a child, I called these periods "living
dreams" because the dreams often continued as I came to
conscious awareness. They would last for moments or what
seemed like hours—the dream images of foreign landscapes, shadows, and figures; they were very "real" even as I
came fully awake.

The memory of my first nightmare is still very clear; it
happened two days after my encounter with the minister.

I am sitting in my living room with my family. A horror movie is playing on the television. Suddenly, I'm

sitting in front of the television. A woman is descending a spiral staircase in an 1890s' gown. She peers over the banister, a look of terror twists her face. There begins a loud, discordant banging on a piano. The sound builds to a crescendo. As the woman puts her hands to her ears, I cover my own ears as the sound intensifies. The sound itself, if I could ascribe an emotion or condition to it, is damned, condemned—as is its player. I know that discordant, mindless playing will continue without end—forever. I can feel the woman's terror; her face—a rictus of panic and fear—mirrors my own. I reach forward and turn off the television set and begin to crawl to my parents' bedroom. A shrouded figure appears in front of me—I know the figure is dead, yet it has come to me. I crawl through the figure, and my parents are watching the same movie I switched off a moment before. I hear the piano from my parents' television set, see the woman still frozen with terror on the spiral staircase. Her terror again becomes my own.

"I'm afraid," I tell my parents. Their eyes are open—but they neither see nor hear me. I am alone. I scream—and the sound melds with the insane cacophony of the piano. I stand up to walk to my room with the music once again building to a crescendo. It is dark. The television casts no light around my parents' bedroom. I feel my way along angular walls to my room. As I approach my room, I hear my brother screaming, screaming. It is nighttime—but in my room it is darker than night. The terror builds to such a level that I am aware I am dreaming within the dream.

"Just a dream," I whisper to myself as I wake up. "Just a dream." I come fully awake from the dream curled in a fetal ball in my bed. It takes me a minute to realize that I am safe.

It seems to me now that the two elements running through that childhood dream were "fear" and "death." The two became synonymous. I remember feeling as if the dream was a further warning from the minister to behave myself.

Indeed I was frightened! I got out of my bed, clenched my hands in front of me, and began to pray. This act did not alleviate my fears at all because at that time prayer was alien to me. I pleaded to a mysterious God to again forgive my sins. I repeated the prayer of salvation the minister taught me. My promise to do good, I was sure, would keep the bad dreams away.

After I prayed and went back to bed, sleep was a long time coming that night. I lay in the dark and wondered what it was that frightened me so badly. Being a child, of course, the deepest fear was of the unknown.

———

I never did utter a word about my nightmares. I did not tell my parents about them—nor did I recount the story of the minister and my being "saved," and I don't exactly know why.

I must have accepted without question the dark pronouncement by the minister of my precarious state: I was on the crossroads between heaven and hell. I understand now that the minister's overemphasis of the dangers of a life of sin was a scare tactic to keep a little boy on the righteous path. But, oh! at what price salvation. The seeds of fear he planted blossomed later in life as guilt and unworthiness. Also among those blossoms was an inherent fear of death itself—regardless of what came afterward. I had a fear of ending. As a child, I used to hold my breath to try to experience "not breathing"—because the dead don't breathe. I thought I could glimpse what death was like in this manner. Of course, I was seized with panic when I held my breath too long, and so I associated death with panic and fear. Death was a frightening mystery to me, and I didn't know how to talk to anyone about the subject. Worse, as a twelve-year-old boy I didn't have the words to express my fears.

By the time I was thirteen, I turned to a world that would provide the answers I so needed: books. My mother was a voracious reader, and she read to me from the time I was a toddler. I inherited her romance with books, and I determined early that through reading I would chase down the fears of my nights, understand the nature of death, probe the possibilities of heaven and hell, and conquer my nightmares. I would wrestle and fight the minister's words and search and search for the truth of a loving God, the God who said, "Let There Be Light!"

Because my grandparents forbade my mother, when she was growing up, to read books on controversial subjects, she let her own children read whatever they felt they could understand.

From the beginning, my road from inner fear to inner peace was an adventurous one. And, as I would soon discover, sometimes perilous.

———

When I was in junior high, during library hour I would scan through the books at school for volumes on nightmares and dreams. I was driven to find answers—and I read with a vengeance. Although I didn't understand what the more adult volumes were about, I checked them out of the library anyway. I read about nightmares and night terrors. I learned that when I wrote my dreams down, they became less ominous.

3

✦

Someone once said that people don't find books; books find people. I do not believe it was an accident that I happened across the article, "What Happens After Death?" in one of my mother's magazines when I was a junior in high school. The article was an excerpt from Raymond Moody's book, *Life After Life*, one of the first publicized reports of near-death experiences (NDEs). In many ways, that article was a life raft; it gave me the ability to cross an ocean of confused childhood fears. I devoured every word of that article and read the accounts from people who returned from a state of clinical death and had reported what they saw. I was amazed to read that many of these people had no religious background, yet they reported inspiring—sometimes heavenly—events.

At the point of death, when vital signs ceased to register,

these people felt themselves being freed from their bodies, floating so that they could see themselves from above the room. Looking down, they saw doctors and nurses attempting to resuscitate their lifeless bodies. They spoke of a feeling of great peace and quiet joy, even though the scene of their deaths was sometimes grisly. One man saw himself after a car accident, his body thrown through the windshield, one of his legs nearly severed. Floating above this scene, he had no feeling except imminent peace. He was not fearful.

The article detailed accounts in which people were being drawn through a dark tunnel with the sound of bells and chimes, seeing colored, flashing lights, and rapidly being drawn into the presence of a benevolent light—an all-knowing, all-loving light that was keenly aware of every aspect of their lives. In the presence of this light, they reported, they reviewed their past and understood all the answers to life and the universe. Above all, they knew they were loved beyond measure. One man reported that the light "knew and loved every unlovable thing about me!" People in this near-death state felt they were an integral part, not separate from, this light. Even when they reviewed pasts filled with "sin," they knew, above all, that they were forgiven. And it was they who had to forgive themselves for unkind thoughts and acts, as there was nothing condemning or foreboding in this light.

A near-death experience would happen over the course of one to nine minutes. Medical practitioners reported that in many cases individuals were "dead" long enough for the brain to be irreparably damaged from lack of oxygen. Yet, these people miraculously returned, often repeating conversations of the resuscitating teams. I was amazed to read the case of one woman who, while in the out-of-body state, floated over the nurses' station at the hospital and remembered the name of a patient being checked in. When she was revived, she asked the doctor if that patient got checked in all right. The doctor was baffled when he checked with the nurses and confirmed what the woman reportedly "saw." She was, for the record, dead at the time of the patient's admission. Others reported seeing deceased family and friends, meeting them on what they called "the other side." They were all present in this all-knowing, all-loving light.

Could this phenomenon be real? There was *evidence* that supported the validity of near-death experiences. I wondered in my mind if these people, who had come close to death, were fulfilling a divine purpose. In some mysterious way, were these near-death experiences not really accidents at all? Did a chosen few on this earth have this happen to reassure frightened people like me? I read on to discover that many people who experienced this light in the near-death state were of various religious backgrounds. Children experienced them, too. If these things were true, then the light was *all* religions of the world and none at all. This being was not some solemn, bearded specter of the night, brandishing eternal punishment to the sinful or providing heaven for the virtuous. This Light was God—a Force—an Intelligence—a Light of Love.

That day in my junior year of high school something rang *true*—as if part of my deeper self knew all about this Light and unconditional love. I had a feeling I had heard these things before—somewhere.

I took the magazine into the kitchen where my mom was doing the supper dishes and asked her about the article.

" 'Near-what' experiences?" she asked.

I began to explain to her a near-death experience—a person seeing himself or herself above the scene, being drawn through a tunnel at rapid speed, the sound of buzzing or bells, then light. I stopped in mid-sentence—Mom's face paled considerably. She stopped washing dishes and was looking at me strangely.

"Mom?" I asked. "What is it?"

"I—I know that tunnel. The lights. Bells. I've seen it." She was visibly shaken. I put the magazine down.

"Seen what, Mom? What happened?"

"Gosh—I've never told anyone about this except your dad. I was afraid people would think I was nuts." She paused, and I could tell from her expression that she was *remembering*. Mom said she had been in the hospital giving birth to my brother Jim. She'd been in labor for some time and they gave her ether.

"After the ether," Mom said, "I heard this buzzing, and I was moving upward—floating. I looked back and I . . . saw myself lying on the table.

"All the nurses were around me," she continued. "Nothing looked as if it were wrong. Then I heard those bells and buzzing noises—real loud, just like you said. And then this tunnel—it's hard to explain because it was so . . . so different. Anyway, I moved through this tunnel—very fast—and there were flashing lights all around me. They looked like stars. There was a 'whooshing' sound in that tunnel—like wind. Then in front of me a lot of people were standing around in white. There was some sort of mist shrouding them. I couldn't see their faces. It felt as though I were there too early—as if it were all premature or something. And when they spoke, they all seemed to be talking at once.

"I don't know, this is crazy!" She was upset by the memory.

I reassured here that literally hundreds of such cases had been reported in Moody's book. The experience was more common than anyone had imagined. I encouraged her to finish the story.

"Anyway, these people in white said, 'How does it feel to be dead?' And they were talking all at once—like one voice."

Despite my comfort with what I had just read, I was shocked. Mom's story sounded worse than my nightmares, but she said the people just seemed concerned.

"And I knew I was giving birth to your brother Jim. I knew

that *over there*. Like I said, it felt too early. And I told them I didn't want to be . . . dead—that I needed to get back. And they said . . . " Her voice trailed off for a moment. "They said, 'You can go back. But you'll never forget what it feels like to be dead.'"

I tried to remain calm. "Mom, you had a near-death experience!"

My mother shook her head. "Well—I don't think I was dead," she said. "The nurses said I took a nice little nap—and that nothing was wrong. My vital signs were fine."

I asked her if the experience seemed like a dream.

"No," she said. "Definitely *not* a dream. It was real. More vivid than a dream."

A lot of people had reported the same feeling during a near-death experience—that their awareness seemed more vibrant; they were more "alive" over there than here on earth. My mother had never spoken of the experience except to my father. Dad believed something had happened to Mom, but they just assumed it was a weird reaction to the ether. Dr. Moody wrote later in his book that often drugs induce an out-of-body or near-death experience.

"It was a strange feeling," Mom said. "After I came home from the hospital, whenever I thought about the experience—it seemed that it was going to come back. I felt as if I was on the verge of it again. As though I could almost feel the tunnel again."

I asked my mother the most important question—to me—about her experience:

"Did it have an effect on what you thought of life after death?"

"We definitely survive death," Mom said. "I know that much for sure."

I was assigned to do a ten-minute speech in English class. I decided to do it on the magazine article about near-death experiences.

Mom cautioned me not to talk about her experience. "People will think you have a crazy family," she said. Her response was exactly like the ones the people in *Life After Life* reported. Many people discussed the experience only with intimate family members. Yet, I could tell Mom felt a lot better for having told me about it. I felt a lot better for hearing it; I knew I was onto something. I silently pledged to become an expert on the subject.

My desire to learn more about the nature of near-death experiences and the nature of death itself became nearly an obsession. The money I saved from mowing lawns was spent on books. The first book was *Life After Life*. One theme ran through nearly all of these cases: People returned without fearing death. They knew death was not the end—that it was merely a passage, a doorway to another, brighter world.

My interest deepened in metaphysical subjects. I frequently visited Waldenbooks in Indianapolis. The occult/mystical section of the bookstore was small, but it contained everything I could want. I was astounded to read books written by "mediums," people who communicated with those who had died. They reported many, diverse worlds outside the physical realm or what they called "the earth plane." The other dimensions were similar to ours—souls went on to other activities; there were schools, "masters" who taught from the realms of "higher learning." Many souls acted as guides for the living. Amazing. Heavenly or hellish states seemed to be individual. Similar to the earth, where all kinds of people live all kinds of lives. I did know people who had heavenly lives; and those who, despondent and disillusioned with life, led hellish ones.

I learned from my reading that where we are in consciousness here on earth is carried over to the next realm. Life continued.

One day, while I was reading in my room with a slew of

metaphysical books on the floor, my dad came in.

"What are you reading now?" he asked.

"Just some other-worldly stuff, Dad. Life after death material." My father was very down to earth, pragmatic. He taught industrial arts in the high school I attended in Morgan. I didn't know what he would think of the subjects; I guessed he would think I was off in left field somewhere.

"Hmmm. It looks . . . interesting," he said, picking up *Here and Hereafter* by Ruth Montgomery. "If you're interested in this kind of stuff," he said, "you ought to read about Edgar Cayce."

I put down the book I was reading. "Who is Edgar Cayce?"

"Edgar Cayce was a psychic," he replied. Hearing my dad say the word *psychic* struck me as funny. I never would have believed he knew about things "other-worldly."

"Cayce could diagnose people's sicknesses and tell them how to get better. He did it in his sleep," Dad said.

"In his sleep?" I asked. "How did he do that?"

"He'd go to sleep, somebody would give him the name and address of a patient who needed help, and Cayce would tell that person how to get well. He never remembered a word of it—and he didn't know anything about medicine, until he went to sleep. If people followed his advice, they got better."

"Wow!" I said. "Where did you hear about this guy?"

"I read a book about him while I was in college in Terre Haute. A guy I worked with swore by Cayce. Said his kids never got colds or the flu because he followed Cayce's health advice."

My dad was usually a man of few words. At least at that point in my life he *seemed* to be. This was a side of him I had never known, but I was delighted.

Edgar Cayce. Sounded like an ordinary name. "I'll check him out, Dad."

"Do that!" he exclaimed. "I don't know about this other

stuff you're reading—but the Cayce stuff is what you ought to be reading, if you want to know about psychics." He smiled and left the room.

In the course of a few short months, I discovered my practical, down-to-earth parents knew about some extraordinary things. My folks, from the rural heartland of America, were "new age." I couldn't believe it.

———

Unfortunately, I didn't immediately take my dad's advice and read up on Edgar Cayce. Instead, I continued to delve into other fantastic and phenomenal psychic stories and experiences.

My quest to understand the nature of my life and where we went at death would take me through some perilous adventures and a myriad of transitions before I reached a coherent understanding of myself in relationship to God. The writing of my experiences today is, itself, a miraculous thing. One of the experiences I passed through nearly ended my life.

4

◆

I experienced a living nightmare when I was sixteen years old. My own curiosity took me down a perilous path that nearly killed me. I went with my friends to a rock concert, and we all purchased LSD. I had read about the mind-expanding drug and knew that LSD was very powerful and unpredictable. I didn't let my naïveté stand in my way. I recklessly took a double dose at the concert and totally lost control.

I settled into my seat at the concert arena, next to five of my closest friends. The visual hallucinations began happening thirty minutes after I took the LSD. The experience was very unusual, but I felt elated. My elation quickly dissipated as the LSD experience gained mental momentum. Soon colors were exploding in front of my eyes. The music had dissolved into a din of confusion. Within an hour of taking the LSD I lost my sense of identity. I didn't know if I was dreaming or awake. The experience seemed to intensify or come in "waves." Each wave brought more confused images and sounds. I found myself in a state of panic.

I can remember blindly running through the packed concert hall, knocking past people who looked like monsters. The last thing I remember, before consciousness slipped away, was pushing my way through the crowd, looking for a door. I was screaming for help but couldn't hear my own words. In the midst of my running, my field of vision went red—a crimson red, like the light in a photographer's darkroom. Everything—the people, the music, the atmosphere, the reality—froze.

When semi-consciousness returned, some four hours later, I was in a parking lot several blocks from the arena. The temperature was zero degrees, but I felt warm. I can remember a floating sensation. I was still heavily under the influence of the LSD at this point, but I have a vivid memory of the following events:

Floating in that semi-conscious state, I looked around myself and could see a platform or stage far, far below me. Somebody was falling into one car after the other in the parking lot on this stage. He was trying to walk but couldn't get balanced. I didn't recognize the stumbling man. He looked like a bum; there were no shoes on his feet, and his pants were torn. I didn't like this scene. I didn't want to see this.

I tried to orient myself to my surroundings, but everything looked foreign. Again and again I was drawn to watch the bum fall down in the parking lot. He looked so cold, and I wondered why nobody would help him.

Then a feeling of dread came over me as I continued to watch the pathetic scene below me. The dread felt like *déjà vu*, as if I were about to experience something dreadful. At that point, the bum stopped falling down and looked up in my direction, high above the parking lot. He craned his head to look up at me. He was *looking at me. Me looking at me.* I was in a state of horror when I realized it was my *body* in the parking lot. That was I!

I felt a movement like an elevator and heard the sound of machinery moving. I was being propelled downward through a tunnel toward the parking lot. From this unusual vantage point I could see myself as others see me. I looked totally different than what I imagined. I saw myself everyday in a mirror, but that really wasn't the true picture at all. This certainly was.

I descended closer and closer to myself in the parking lot, feeling panic-stricken. There was a sound of buzzing, bells, something like half-voices which were calling, directing, lamenting. Then I was face to face with myself. In the moment that I descended from somewhere out-of-body, my life was surrounding me—every thought, deed, and experience. But it was all the *wrong* things. The bad things: the accidents, mishaps, and disappointments. Through that tunnel with the lights and bells and buzzing was my life, but I could only see the dark side of it. The scenes kept repeating and going on, in one simultaneous moment. No end or beginning.

Hell. This is hell.

Then the sounds and bells stopped. The panoramic view of life scenes stopped just as I experienced a flash of light and the sensation of "placement"—my mind joining my body. I felt the weight of my body; it was so *heavy.* I opened my eyes and was shocked to find myself looking into the direction from which I had just come. I screamed—thinking this to be the worst nightmare of my life: I had become the bum in the parking lot. Looking down, I was horrified to see I indeed had no shoes on. My jeans were torn.

I thought that this experience *was* a dream. Especially when I checked my watch and saw the digital readout: *1:33 a.m.* All of the bizarre events became too much for my conscious mind to handle, and once again I felt that "click" or switch of consciousness shut off. I passed out. For how long, I don't know, but eventually I was being shaken awake.

"Rob, wake up." It was a familiar voice. I opened my eyes. A man was standing in front of me. He had thin, red hair, wire-frame glasses, and a black jacket with an American flag on the sleeve. He knew my name.

"You know me?" I said. My voice sounded strange and echoed.

"I've always known you."

Dread. *What in God's name was happening to me?* "Who are you?" I asked.

He smiled at me. "Come on. I'll buy you a coke."

"No. I don't want to go with you."

After the experience I had just been through, I was convinced I was no longer in the world as I knew it. This couldn't be my world, because this strange man knew my name. I distrusted him immediately.

"No," I said again, "I'm not going."

"O.K.," the red-haired man said, "suit yourself." He started to walk away.

"Wait!" I cried. Even though I didn't trust him, I didn't trust being alone either. I got to my feet. "Help me." I felt so *lost.*

The man looked at me patiently. "Why did you take the LSD?" he asked.

How did he know what I took? How did he know my name?

"I—it was a mistake—I didn't think about it. Everybody did it." I tried to think of a good reason for taking LSD and made a feeble attempt. "I wanted to expand my mind. Please tell me who you are and how you know me."

"You can call me Bill." His voice was pleasant, and he seemed compassionate. "And I've always known you."

"No. I don't know you—you're not real." I started to cry, feeling a million miles from home. God, I couldn't remember how I got here in this place! I remembered the concert—and the awfulness—and it still felt bad, really bad. I missed my mom and dad. I felt as if I would never see them again.

"Oh, please help me," I cried. "Please get me home."

"I can't do that," Bill said, shaking his head. "But somebody will help you. Come on."

Still crying, I looked around the parking lot that I didn't remember arriving at; I looked at this man who knew me, but whom I never knew. I was stuck. Where I was stuck, I had no idea. Feeling hopeless and helpless, I followed this man. I wondered where my shoes were. I felt the cold rocks under my feet. I reached for my wallet. It, too, was missing. My identity was gone. My belt was even missing.

"My God, mister," I pleaded, "what has happened to me? Where am I?"

I was in hysterics. Bill held onto my arm and led me to a warehouse office. He opened an industrial door and sat me in a chair outside a small office. He quickly dialed from a telephone—watching me all the while. I silently prayed for deliverance.

———

As I closed my eyes to pray, I slipped into unconsciousness. I awoke when a uniformed policeman was shaking me.

"Come on, son," he said. The policeman looked to be in his late fifties, gray hair. I looked into his eyes. He looked dismayed—just like Bill had looked. It was as though everybody knew my precarious state of mind.

"Where's Bill?" I asked, getting to my feet.

"Who's Bill?" the policeman asked suspiciously, looking around the warehouse with his flashlight.

"He called you," I replied. "He said he would help me."

"No one called me, kid. Come on, let's go."

I was confused. "But—Bill called you—he said—"

"Kid, the warehouse door was open; it's never open this time of night. Come on. You have the right to remain silent." The policeman handcuffed me and began reading me my rights!

I protested and pleaded with the police officer that there had been some mistake. Finally I asked him what I had done wrong.

"Looks to me like breaking and entering. Plus you're stoned out of your mind, kid. Why don't you just keep quiet. You're under arrest. You have the right to have an attorney present ... "

He put me in the back of the police car and took me to Wishard Memorial Hospital in downtown Indianapolis. I faded in and out of consciousness during the ride. I vaguely remember driving past Market Square Arena en route to the hospital. *How had I gotten to that warehouse?*

I again felt consciousness slipping away, but I was no longer afraid. Whoever or whatever Bill was, the last thought I had was the realization that Bill *had* helped me. He was something like my guardian angel. He had intervened for me. The thought was clear and lucid—and I fell asleep.

———

How close did I come to losing it all? Losing my life? Given the paranormal events surrounding my experience, I would say I came very, very close to death. I remember that strange place where all the bad things of my life happened and repeated. I had seen hell. Yet, I had been given a second chance, it seems, at life. I knew I had traveled to the brink of death and somehow had been allowed to come back.

It wasn't until I read Raymond Moody's follow-up book to *Life After Life—Reflections on Life After Life*—that I understood I had had a near-death experience. I was reading the chapter on suicide—and I felt a chilling sense of *déjà vu* as I read Dr. Moody's comments—as well as the individual's comments about her near-death experience:

> "One person mentioned being 'trapped' in the situation which had provoked her suicide attempt. She had the feeling that the state of affairs in which she had been before her 'death' was being repeated again and again, as if in a cycle.
>
> " 'This problem I was telling you about, you know, well, looking back on it now, of course, it doesn't seem so important, from a more adult way of looking at it. But at the time, as I was a person at that age, it really seemed very important . . . Well, the thing was, it was still around, even when I was "dead." And it was like it was repeating itself, a rerun. I would go through it once and at the end I would think, "Oh, I'm glad that's over," and then it would start all over again, and I would think, "Oh, no, not this again." ' "

Reading this account brought home the surety of how close to death I had come. Even though the LSD trip was not a suicide attempt, the state of consciousness I entered was one that put me in a state of "death" by my own hand. People who had NDEs through accidents reported all the *good* events of their lives, happening simultaneously. My experience was opposite, just as the woman's who attempted suicide.

Another aspect of my experience I have wondered about: Who was Bill? I even went back months later to the warehouse where I was found to see if there were any employees named Bill. No one fit the name or the description.

Many people reported in their NDEs that there were guides and guardians, angelic beings who knew all about them and their lives. I can't help but feel that this Bill was my guardian.

This adverse LSD experience left me with an assurance that I am indeed guided—guarded—even in the most precarious of situations. Since that experience, I have many times felt the assurance that I would make it through the difficult periods in my life.

Although the LSD experience was by far one of the most frightening things that's ever happened to me, out of it was born a sense that there is a purpose to my being here now, and it deepened my belief in a caring, protective Creator—even in moments when I was carelessly reckless. I found it to be true that, as the Bible said, we often entertain angels unaware. I have no doubt that one of them guided me back to my life on earth.

5
◆

*W*hen I remember the Indiana of my youth, there is a convergence of different senses: I smell the coming of spring out of the last remnants of winter; I see our home from a bird's-eye view, like a Norman Rockwell painting; I hear the sounds of birds; I smell the harvested corn in October; I feel both vast and lonely. The appearance of the rural woodlands of Indiana are indeed like the works of Wyeth or Rockwell—brilliant colors, spacious hills and skies, cornfields. The rural country where I was born is beautiful in spring and autumn; the winters long, dreary, and cold. As a child, I would anxiously await the coming of spring to take away the gray and overcast skies of the Indiana winter. Sunlight was a precious commodity from November to March. The absence of the sun made the winter landscape gloomy, barren, desolate. Then there are the colors of gray and winter and isolation. It is the contrast of the very best and the very worst, the very light and very dark. In the remembrance of my years in Indiana I felt those same contrasts.

Our home in Morgan was nestled in several acres of secluded woodlands—unseen and unchanged by the progress of modern life. Our house was situated on a hill overlooking Highway 67. Across the two-lane highway we could see the banks and currents of White River.

On the six acres of woodlands my parents bought in 1960, my older brothers and I were raised in the nostalgic traditions of my mother and father. Although I grew up in the 1960s and '70s, it could have been the 1940s. The years were timeless because my folks did not keep up with modern traditions as the outside world progressed.

My mother, a teacher by profession and homemaker by choice, devoted her life to raising her family. When many women of America were heading to professional lives outside the home, she was content to continue homemaking as her life's work. My mother would only smile when asked by friends and relatives, "Mary Lou, your kids are all in school [at this time John was in sixth grade, Jim was in fourth, I was in second]—when are you going to go back to 'work'?"

When I became a teen-ager, I would jump to the defense of my mother's decision to remain a professional homemaker. I don't remember a day when she was not up by 6:00 every morning. She made homemaking a divine art. My grandmother taught her to cook in her pre-teen years. By the time I was born she had mastered cooking and was preparing culinary masterpieces.

Our dinners together were a ritual: It was a time when the entire family came together to celebrate being a family. I was expected to be home for the evening meal by 5:30 p.m. This wasn't a bendable rule—it was important to my mother and father to have structured and set times where we were all together as a family. When growing up, my father didn't have the luxury of having enough to eat. Most of the time he and his sister fended for themselves at mealtime. When he raised a family, he made sure there would be food in abundance. Although he was raising a family of five on the income of a high school teacher, we never went without.

Looking back at the daily living of my growing years, I can see that my father and mother led diverse and separate lives during the working day. Dad taught machine shop at the local high school. During his time off, he was building additions to the house, laying cement, fixing cars. My mother cleaned our home, washed our clothes, baked dazzling desserts, cooked our meals, planted brilliantly colored flowers and plants outside our home, tamed the wildlife that lived on our property: squirrels, raccoons, chipmunks—even snakes. The woodland creatures overran our property. Mom got in the habit of calling them "pushy wildlife," especially when squirrels and chipmunks would sit on the window sill and eat out of the bird feeders.

My mother and father passed one another through their days together. Meals were the times they shared their experiences of the days. Yet it wasn't uncommon for me to come home from bike riding in the summertime and see Mom up on the roof pounding nails, reshingling the roof with Dad, or she would be helping him take the motor out of a car in the garage. Dad was also very good around the house. Every Saturday night my folks cooked homemade pizza. Dad created the recipe himself and would make the dough from scratch. My parents were a great complement to one another and they took a great deal of interest in each other's professions.

After years of "sharing professions," my mother became excellent in diagnosing automotive problems. Dad was always proud of the fact that he had never spent more than $500 on a car or truck. This was true even in 1979 when I was a senior in high school. He would rebuild the engines, do bodywork, and repaint. We usually had four or five cars and trucks in various stages of completion on the property.

By the same token, Dad could talk recipes with Mom and he loved being in the kitchen. He would whip up unusual dishes. Dad was always good about giving Mom what he called "helpful hints" for better cooking. We always laughed a lot over Dad's gourmet ideas. More times than not, Mom would shoo him out of the way and send him back out to his garage or his metalworking shop.

My parents had the rare and precious gift of being best friends as well as husband and wife; they had been together since their junior year of high school. They had even been prom sweethearts.

We were a close family in many ways. We talked about books, television, politics, the arts. The greatest discussions that ever took place were during supper. But rarely did we discuss feelings and emotions. This is where I felt a world apart from my parents and older brothers. My oldest brother John had inherited my father's gift of being able to repair and fix anything mechanical. My middle brother, Jim, took to the building trades and worked construction during his high school years. I was the most introspective of the family, fascinated with books and the arts. I always felt a bit out of place, a stranger to our rustic way of life. Yet, I loved this wilderness and the enchanted surrounding woodlands.

6

◆

*T*he acres of forest surrounding my home became a world alive, full of wonder and adventurous possibilities. The best of my growing-up years were spent exploring the mysteries of nature. I would run through the woodland trails that my brothers and I had made, leaping over the patches of May apples, climbing the aged oaks and hickory trees. Mushroom hunting was an annual spring tradition in Morgan, Indiana—and I would search for hours for those elusive delicacies, usually hidden under leaves near the stumps of fallen trees. After soaking the mushrooms in salt water for a day (to get the bugs out), my mother would batter and fry them as a side dish for supper. Every year in March and April the whole family would set out for the woods to go mushroom hunting. Particularly in Morgan was this considered a community sport. I enjoyed those family outings, but I relished the time apart where the only voices I heard were the voices of nature.

I was alone in many of my forest explorations, but only in body. There were nature spirits abounding in the woods. Although I could not see them, I spoke aloud to them. After reaching adulthood, I attributed my communion with the nature spirits to a vivid imagination. I found it interesting that in *There Is a River*, Thomas Sugrue's biography of Edgar Cayce, there was much discussion about the nature spirits. I was amazed to learn that, as a child, Edgar Cayce could see the nature gnomes and fairies. Edgar's mother could also see them, and she would often tell him that "his friends" were waiting for him to come out and play. Cayce even gave readings on the nature spirits and called them "elementals." As an adult, he would often tell stories about his friendship with the miniature spirit beings whom he called "the little folk."

"Anyone can see them," Cayce once said. "However, to see them you have to have the mind of a child and believe in them." I was amazed! My imaginary friends hadn't been imaginary at all. Years later I read a passage in one of the psychic "readings" that Cayce gave that made me feel special: Anyone who understands nature walks closely with God. I felt the closest to this natural God while in the woods during the month of October at the height of Indian summer, when the woods exploded in brilliant colors. As a child, I was definitely aware of a majestic presence all around me in my woodland explorations. I know of no better religious experience than the view of nature at the height of autumn. As a small boy, I considered this my religion: The hills were my sacred sanctuary, the trails were mysterious paths leading to uncharted territory, the songs of the locusts were choirs of angels. I worshiped daily in this temple with no walls or doors, created by a divine Architect that human hands could never replicate.

My favorite place was a fallen hickory tree that formed a bridge across a gully with a massive beech tree nearby. Hearts and names and dates were carved into the tree. I often ran my hand across the months and years that predated my birth. I felt so young in comparison to the mammoth tree. The large oaks, hickories, and beeches stood like ancient protectorates, guardians, silent friends. There were moments when I could almost feel the forest as a thing alive. The songs of a hundred birds, the winds, and the locusts all converged in nature's symphony. I would crane my head back and see the tops of trees swaying as if in response to the music of nature. I felt happy and safe there in my woods. Although I often felt lonely during my days in school, in nature I was wrapped in her companionship much too vast for the limitations of loneliness.

The woods and the sanctuary I found there were never far from my awareness—and their memory kept me warm.

7

◆

N ew ideas, feelings, thoughts, and questions swirled in my mind, especially after the LSD experience. In moments when I was doing mundane chores around the house or bicycling or reading, it was as if my mind had become opened to some sort of inquisitive wavelength that asked universal questions. I had an inner desire and urge to know myself at a deeper level. I needed to look at my life, to know from where I came and where I was going. I wondered why couldn't I simply live my life without questioning, as so many people seemed to do? Why was it so important for me to grasp something so intangible and elusive? What if the reports of near-death experiences were right? At the point of death would there be a review of the life I had lived from a broadened fourth-dimensional view? What would my life look like? I imagined (or hoped) what I thought of as "good" and "bad" experiences would not be viewed in such a limited perspective as good and evil, heaven and hell.

I thought perhaps that when life was completed, it would reflect a mosaic, painted full and beautiful with experiences: The shadows, the negatives of life, made the lighter moments seem brighter. If there was no shadow, how could the brilliance of light be seen? I could see myself—here, in this life—being so critical of my sins, faults, and weaknesses, rarely giving credit to myself; then passing to a realm uninhibited by earthly limitations and condemnation, a realm that used love as the measure of how well life was lived. I tried to imagine what the experience would be like to see my life before me—panoramic as one brilliant moment or event in time.

In this three-dimensional world I could see that earthly life is portrayed by religion as a struggle between good and evil. Perhaps from the Creator's viewpoint each life is but a dance of the light with the dark.

The LSD episode—as frightening as it was—had certainly broadened my perspective of consciousness. Having come close to losing my life, I felt that the experience deepened my search to understand the nature of life and death. My studies did take me into the work of Edgar Cayce. It began with a book, *Meditation—One Step Beyond with Edgar Cayce*. I discovered what people of the Eastern religions had believed for thousands of years: The path to truly understanding ourselves, God, life, and death is within.

The first time I sat down to meditate, I followed the directions outlined in the book. As I sat quietly, I did a series of breathing exercises, said the Lord's Prayer, chanted, and repeated words that would attune my mind to the meditative state. As my mind began to wander (just as the book said it would), I easily brought my focus back with the words, *God is Love. Love is God.* I repeated these words in my head as often as my mind wandered.

After some minutes, I became aware that my mind was silent. Not silent in the sense of an absence of words, but I was enveloped in an active quietude—a feeling—a place—The Silence. It was not alarming. I felt as if I had risen slightly from where I was sitting and was on a shelf or a cliff—and this place was filled with this "active silence." I became acutely aware that most of the time my mind was filled with a kind of background noise. I noticed this because now in this state there was no mental noise at all. I marveled at the peace that accompanied the silence. I could feel that my mind had never been this silent, never been this calm. I felt that I traveled to a definite place. Then, there came a thought, a feeling, an experience: *All Is Well.*

These words were a living concept—I was an integral part of it. I was quiet and reverent within the awakening. This, a part of my mind reasoned, was God. I knew this in the way one knows it's summer or spring. The awareness was fact within my psyche: This silence was the abode of the Divine Source or God. The experience expanded, and in startled realization I knew that I was a vital part of this Force that proclaimed, *All Is Well.* This reality reverberated all through my body and mind. I knew myself, as well as all other people, to be an eternal part of this Being and that I never would be separate from It. I knew that this Being was cognizant of my small self and my minute part of the universe. There was immense joy in this knowing. How seasoned and old I felt! Not old in the sense of time, but in experience. I was beyond my physical age of sixteen, yet I was an ageless being. The boundaries and limitations of physical time didn't seem to touch my soul. I was not a being of years; I was a season—moving, changing, shifting, and growing. I felt as if I had always been conscious.

Before this meditation, I had thought of eternity as a solemn, never-ending experience to be endured. In the midst of this calmness of spirit, I knew eternity to be the length and scope of my real self. Eternity wasn't out there as some place—it was an event, an activity, a moment. It was also me. Me! I felt the full comprehension of myself as a soul, a traveler, an adventurer. The joy resided in the full realization that I was known by a power, a force, a Creator greater than I could imagine.

All of this didn't seem strange at all to my young mind. I had no words for the experience—it was natural and yet new at the same time. With a sense of relief I knew this Force did not see the darkness of my sins, but the light of my soul.

The experience gradually faded, and I remembered the book said to pray for others at the close of meditation. I prayed a prayer of thanks for the feelings of great peace and then repeated the Twenty-third Psalm, which I had learned years before in grade school. As I opened my eyes, I was still filled with the Silence. I promised myself to return every day.

Of one thing I was sure, there was no darkness or evil in this Being. Hell was no part of this all-loving, serene Force. I seemed to know that hell was humankind's creation: If individuals willed themselves into hellish circumstances, that is where they would find themselves. What people willed, God could not prevent. But there was intervention for humankind's recklessness. This took many forms—in the way of angels or guides or guardians. I read in this book on meditation that each of us has a definite guide or guardian who is assigned to each soul. There's a biblical passage that verifies this truth: "He shall give his angels charge concerning thee . . . lest at any time thou dash thy foot against a stone." (Matthew 4:6)

I had more than dashed my foot in the past; and I was beginning to understand that a force we call God was most aware of my predicaments and had provided some form of divine intervention. Yet, if I were to believe the fundamentalist minister—the minister who found me at age twelve—he would have me believe that God abandons those who are foolhardy in their indulgent and "sinful" activities—not only are they abandoned, they are sent to suffer eternal torment. I knew, in my heart, after this meditative experience, that this was no part of that Creative Force. I felt sad that the minister did not have this knowing that God was infinitely kind. I imagined also that God, the Force Itself, was perhaps a bit sad that this minister had painted such a grim picture of Him.

———

As I delved more deeply into the psychic readings of Edgar Cayce, I became more fascinated. The amazing part of the story is that Cayce would awaken from one of these "reading" periods and say, "Did we get it?" When people who requested Cayce's readings acknowledged that indeed they did receive helpful information, Cayce's usual reply was "Thank God." He attributed his unusual gift to God and vowed that, as long as people got well, he would give readings. Yet, acceptance of his gift was a lifelong struggle for him. His secretary, Gladys Davis, who transcribed the readings word for word as they were given, said that Cayce constantly had to be reassured that his ability was worthwhile and that people were indeed being helped. He worried that he might prescribe a dangerous remedy that would do great harm. Cayce said on more than one occasion that if anyone got hurt by the information, he would give it up.

No one got hurt, but thousands of people got well by following his advice. I learned that more than 8,000 people came to Cayce for advice on all kinds of subjects. At some point people concluded that if Cayce could diagnose an illness in a person he'd never met or seen, then he might be able to answer some of the questions that have been puzzling humankind throughout time. Not only did he answer universal questions, Cayce gave dissertations on the nature of God and the destination of the soul. He also gave an interpretation of the Book of Revelation. He gave readings on the creation, the story of Adam and Eve. He interpreted dreams and believed that dreams were to be utilized in everyday living for guidance. He spoke of the future and gave prophecies through the end of the twentieth century. The metaphysical readings were amazing, but the majority—two-thirds—of readings dealt with the healing of disease.

One of the most remarkable concepts I found in the Cayce readings was the idea of "the one God," that all people, races, and religions are an integral part of one Force or God. All life, in its diverse forms, emanated from one Source. It seemed to me that this One Creative Force had great variety in Its creations—hence, the innumerable world religions and beliefs. The readings said that all religions could be summarized in what Jesus said two thousand years ago:

Love God, and love your neighbor as yourself. (Matthew 22:37, 39)

So where did I fit into all of this? Before I had read about Cayce, I had felt as if I stumbled upon a stage where my life was being played out in a sea of circumstances beyond my control. In my unfolding awareness, as I studied the concepts in Cayce's material, I was beginning to see that life was purposeful and maybe even divine. In our journey through earth life, I began to accept that we are all living our own examples of what we believe God to be. In our thoughts, deeds, and activities, I felt we either exemplified or desecrated our concept of God. It made life, for me, a sort of cosmic drama. We, as Shakespeare had said, were not only players on the world's stage, but also the writers, producers, and directors. It was all within our control. The vastness of these concepts and ideas overwhelmed me, yet it made the inevitability of my own death a small thing. The survival of the soul at physical death was a certainty, according to the Cayce readings. In the readings I found what I so badly wanted to believe was true: We always have been and we always will be. Eternity is not some place in the hereafter, it is an experience. It is now.

While I was reading *On Death and Dying* by Elisabeth Kübler-Ross, I could understand her concept that we should not fear death, rather we should fear not living life to the fullest *today.*

I graduated from high school in 1979. It was with a great relief that my preliminary education was over. It felt like the end of a great battle.

After graduation I thought back to my childhood with many fond memories. I also thought of the fundamentalist minister who proclaimed damnation and hellfire warnings to me at such a young age. Did I need this experience so that I would search more deeply in this life? Was I driven out of fear to find answers? If so, perhaps I was doing well—I *was* searching. And I was finding as well.

My traditional education paled in comparison to what I had learned about the nature of life. I did not have many answers, but I felt I had made progress on the road to understanding the nature of life and God, and the role I was playing in it. As always there were the paradoxical feelings that I was so young and yet so old at the same time. Another paradox was feeling how much I had learned and yet how little I knew.

The season came when I knew it was time to move on. My departure from the rural hills of Middle America was to be a great change. In many ways it was like a death; I was leaving the familiar spaces and places on a journey into the unknown. Most of my friends had left for college, gotten married, or were working in mundane jobs in Morgan. I, too, had been working a mundane job in a warehouse in Indianapolis. Something restless in me had awakened; I yearned to see the east and west coasts, Europe, the Holy Land.

I shuddered at the thought of college. I couldn't see myself going to war again with textbooks and classes. I wanted to experience a real education. I wanted to learn from the world and its mysteries. I didn't want to read history; I longed to see it, experience it, and feel myself a part of it. The best way I knew to experience the world was to join the navy. It was not a new idea in my family; Dad and my two older brothers had spent four years in the navy. None had made it a career, but they enjoyed the travel.

I went to Indianapolis to be inducted. My indoctrination into navy life was not as much of a shock as I had anticipated. I adapted well, even to boot camp at the training center in Great Lakes, Illinois. No doubt my structured and regimented upbringing had a lot to do with my ability to adapt to the military. I faced the changes with little fear; there were eighty other guys in my company who were just as new to this as I.

The days went by quickly.

A remarkable thing happened the day I received my duty station orders: Nearly everyone was assigned to report to sea duty aboard a ship; I was one of three people who got assigned two years of shore duty at the naval air station in Norfolk, Virginia. After two weeks' leave in Indiana, I was to report for duty at an aviation squadron.

During my two-week stay at home, I was given a present by Lois Bennett, a friend who shared my spiritual quest. The gift was in the form of a book called *Illusions* (Delacorte Press/Eleanor Friede, 1977) by Richard Bach. As I was reading about a "reluctant messiah" (he was as gifted as Jesus, but he didn't care for crowds), I came across a passage that spoke of the wondrous aspects of change and transition:

> "You are led through your lifetime by the inner learning creature, the playful spiritual being that is your real self. Don't turn away from possible futures before you're certain you don't have anything to learn from them . . . In order to live free and happily, you must sacrifice boredom. It is not always an easy sacrifice."

For me, boredom was the prospect of remaining in Indiana and being fearful of the outside world. In many of my friends' eyes, I had taken a great leap into the unknown by joining the navy. I saw my friends' boredom, their fear of change, and their clinging to the mundane. Bach was right, I thought. After being entrenched in a familiar life, it was difficult to have faith, step out, and take a chance. Yet, if I believed that I was essentially a spiritual being who came to learn that, no matter what road I traveled, I would always be taken care of when I took chances or risks, I had learned in the short period of my life a valuable lesson: I had discovered God in the stormy nights of unsureness and fear. Now in the new phase of my life, I realized that no matter where I went or what passages and changes I would endure, that Voice would always be with me proclaiming *All Is Well.* In that light, boredom was very easy to sacrifice indeed.

8

✦

N orfolk, Virginia, proved to be a valuable part of my spiritual journey. I had the opportunity to talk with Hugh Lynn Cayce, Edgar Cayce's son, every Friday for several months. Norfolk was only twenty miles from Virginia Beach, where Edgar Cayce and a small group of his supporters had established a teaching and research organization in the early 1930s. Named the Association for Research and Enlightenment, Inc., the nonprofit organization had established its worldwide headquarters in the Atlantic coast resort city with Hugh Lynn Cayce as its president, who continued to examine and expand his father's work. My meeting resulted from a letter I wrote to him about my childhood fears of death and my nightmares and night terrors. I also wanted to understand what had happened to me during the LSD incident and the unusual state of consciousness I awoke to. Hugh Lynn had written a book, *Venture Inward,* in the early 1960s. In it, he discussed hallucinogens. I had asked him detailed questions in my letter and was excited by the handwritten note I received from him several days later:

"Dear Rob,
"My secretary is in Egypt, hence this written note. Let's talk. Here's my telephone number at work and at home. Give a call next week and set up an appointment. Fridays are open.
"See you soon, Hugh Lynn."

Edgar Cayce's son wanted to see *me*? I was astounded. What an opportunity! It seemed it was no accident that my work schedule at the squadron happened to be Monday through Thursday. Fridays were free, too.

I was twenty at the time, and it had been four years since the LSD experience. I had the feeling that I would find many answers to my questions at the A.R.E. But I never imagined I would get a chance to ask questions of the son of Edgar Cayce. I knew that Hugh Lynn had taken up the study of his father's psychic work as his own life's mission. He was the foremost authority on virtually all topics in the Cayce readings.

The first Friday came, and I took the scenic route on Shore Drive to the Cayce headquarters at the oceanfront. The last several miles to the Association looked like the rural roads of Indiana. It was autumn of 1981, and the leaves on the trees were beginning to turn. The drive brought back the memories of autumn in the woods of my youth. Again I was filled with that sense of well-being I always experience in the wooded hills.

I pulled into the parking lot off Atlantic Avenue and walked up to the old white-framed building on the hill. The building had been the Cayce Hospital in the 1920s, where people could come and be treated by physicians according to Cayce's readings.

I walked into Hugh Lynn's office, where his secretary greeted me. "He'll be right with you. Just have a seat."

I took a seat in the outer office. I noticed a portrait of Jesus hanging on the wall.

"Are you Rob?"

I looked up and saw a white-haired gentleman, rather tall, whose eyes twinkled. I guessed he was in his seventies. For some reason, I never imagined Hugh Lynn to be that old. But then, I remembered that Edgar Cayce had died in 1945.

"Yes, I am," I said, extending my hand.

"Come in," he said, shaking my hand. He led me into a modest office and closed the door. "I read your letter. Very interesting. You've got a lot of questions! How old are you, Rob?"

"Twenty."

"For some reason, I thought you'd be older," he said.

"For some reason, I thought you'd be younger," I replied. Our eyes met and we both laughed. "I didn't mean that the way it sounded!" I protested.

"I know, I know," he said still chuckling. He immediately put me at ease. Hugh Lynn was looking over the letter I had written him. I began to talk about the LSD experience and how I couldn't help but believe that I had come near to death.

"Oh, my, did you ever!" Hugh Lynn said. "You're extremely lucky. Some people on drugs who get to that out-of-body state of consciousness never leave it. They're stuck there."

"For how long?" I asked, a little startled.

"Until the physical body dies—even then it may be longer."

"You mean, you've heard of other people having this experience?" I asked.

"Oh, yes. Many times. Taking LSD was quite the rage in the 1960s. Few people realized what a bad trip entailed. One young man stumbled into my office some years ago; he was much in the same state of mind you were. Totally out of it. What I mean is, *totally out of his body*," he said emphatically. "There is what my father called the 'silver cord' that connects the soul to the body. At the point of death, that cord is severed. In the experience you had—and this other boy—the soul is very much 'out there,' but this connection of the silver cord is still intact. When you saw yourself stumbling around in the parking lot from this out-of-body state, you were seeing only the body—without the counterpart of the mind and soul. You were in such an expanded state of consciousness, far removed from the three-dimensional world. That is why you didn't recognize yourself."

"And you say this other guy who was on LSD, you knew he was out of his body?"

"His soul was not in his body. His movements were jerky, not coordinated, and he couldn't speak. It took me hours to get him back in his body."

"How did you do that?" I asked, amazed.

"Prayer, mostly. The power of prayer and some laying-on-of-hands healing. You see, when you take LSD, you open up what my father called the 'spiritual centers' in the body. These centers contain all states of consciousness—all kinds of dimensions. We can experience all that through meditation. But the spiritual centers, or what people of the Eastern philosophies call the 'chakras,' should only be opened naturally, so that the experience of other dimensions doesn't come crashing into us, like what happened to you."

I was trying to digest all of this.

"When you take LSD," Hugh Lynn added, "you might as well have taken a blowtorch to your spiritual centers—it just burns them open. The reason people have 'flashbacks,' a recurrence of the hallucinogenic state, is that their centers will open spontaneously and project them back into the altered state of consciousness. Even after the LSD experience is over, the centers can open any time. Usually, they're like sealed doors, but hallucinogens burn that seal off. Like breaking the lock and hinges off a door."

"But isn't the LSD what is causing the experience in the first place?" I asked.

"LSD or mushrooms or anything of the sort is merely a mechanism to heighten the mind's awareness of already existing circumstances and states of consciousness. It's a key to a door or a switch. But most of the time, our three-dimensional consciousness is not ready to handle fourth-, fifth-, or even seventh-dimensional experiences."

Hugh Lynn leveled his eyes at me. "Everything you experienced under LSD was very real. It's not an hallucination. And let me tell you, there's plenty of things in this universe that you do not *want* to see—as you saw."

"Yes." I shuddered with the memory of it all. My mind was racing. What I had experienced was real. No wonder it seemed so vivid at the time.

"And the conscious mind," Hugh Lynn went on, "is only aware of the you, the personality, right now. When you blast open those spiritual centers like you did, a million images— psychic images, thought forms, and patterns—assaulted your conscious mind, which is not able to stand such things. It was natural that it shut down. Realize, too, that if you were to take any type of hallucinogen again, it could project you right back into that state of mind."

I shuddered again. "I have no intention of doing that again."

"Like I said, you're very lucky. Many people have gouged out their eyes while using psychoactive drugs. What they see is so horrible, they tear out their eyes. I also know of kids who jumped off bridges and buildings under the influence of LSD."

"I know why they do that," I said. "The things that you see and feel—it's just hellish, a nightmare. I don't want to go through that ever again."

"Glad to hear it," he said, smiling, "you've got work to do

here." As I looked into his eyes, he seemed to be seeing something more in me than just a curious young man. It was as though he were gazing into my future. I felt as if I'd known Hugh Lynn Cayce for a long, long time.

"But this Bill guy—what was that all about?" I asked.

Hugh Lynn smiled. "My father said that each and every person on earth has a guardian angel. It may be an extension of yourself, your 'higher self,' or it may be someone who has passed on. We all have guides and guardians."

"He seemed to know everything about me," I said.

"If you were a guardian for someone," he said gently, "wouldn't you know everything about the person you were taking care of?"

"I guess I would."

"Did you ever hear the Bible verse that says, 'God hath given his angels charge concerning thee'?" (Matthew 4:6)

"Yes," I said at once, "I believed it after the LSD experience."

———

The conversations we had over the next five months gave me a sense of direction and a purpose. I felt I was on the right track in my journey toward understanding myself as a soul and was coming close to understanding what my purpose on earth was.

"Knowing these things," Hugh Lynn said on one occasion, "you'll be a great help to a great many people."

I hoped that eventually I would be able to share information as Hugh Lynn shared with me. He taught me so much about the nature of life and of death. I'm sure my questions were elementary to him, but he was patient in his explanations.

On the nature of the death experience, Hugh Lynn told me that the state of consciousness in which we leave this world is the same state in which we will find ourselves after death. No wonder I was projected into a confused state during that near-death experience. I had been in that state while in the body. The consciousness continues. The transition we go through at death is just that: a transition. A change of place. Merely leaving the body behind. Our mental state of being stays the same.

"There are many more difficult experiences a soul or entity will go through in life," Cayce said, "than what you call death.

"Life," he added, "is a continuous experience."

Hugh Lynn told me that our circumstances after death depended greatly upon what was our focus here on earth.

"My father often said we go to the place in consciousness we have created or built for ourselves. It's not permanent, but remember that time isn't the same over there. Dad was in the middle of a reading once and interrupted himself and said: 'This is interesting! The entity known as (he gave a man's name) has been what you call dead for some ten years and has just realized it!' If we strive for only the material life and urges, we'll find ourselves in an earthbound state of consciousness, still hovering in the material world and unable to leave it. A hell indeed!"

"Does the soul ever get out of that hell or is it forever?" This was at the heart of my deepest fears.

Hugh Lynn was very thoughtful for a moment. "Until that soul seeks help, it will stay there. But help is always there. It's just like here on earth. People are often lost in their own worlds, trapped by their own circumstances. Have you ever known people who resist change and stay in miserable situations?"

"Yeah," I agreed. "A lot of my friends back home are bored with their lives. They seem unhappy."

"Exactly the same on the 'other side,' " Hugh Lynn said. "Help in the form of guardian angels and forces are always surrounding that earthbound soul. But it's the soul that must make the decision or awaken itself to move on."

"I don't want to find myself in that state," I said. "What

can I do to make sure I'm free from that state?"

"Meditate," he said. "People don't realize the power in meditation. It has two major benefits: It helps us to attune ourselves to the Infinite or God, and it develops the soul to the point that it is free from the earth at death. People talk about seeing a light in near-death experiences. That's what we're trying to do in meditation, find that light while we're in the body. If we find it here in the physical consciousness, we can be sure we'll find it after death."

Hugh Lynn Cayce believed in reincarnation. But for him it was more than an idea or a concept. It was a living example that we are continuously growing, developing, and becoming aware of our soul selves.

"We are," Hugh Lynn said, during one of our last sessions together, "a sum total of all of our experiences—now. We are everything we have ever been and done. A composite. We change throughout the eons, but we never die. Much in the same way when you turn a light off, the energy or light changes form and becomes invisible to our eyes, but it still exists. The same is for us. As the body dies, the soul—invisible, intangible—changes form and goes on. We are *in* the body; we are *not* the body."

I remembered Charles Dickens's *A Christmas Carol* and thought it to be a brilliant allegory about how we create our own heaven or our own hell in the hereafter. Scrooge goes home on Christmas Eve and the ghost of his old business partner, Marley, appears. He is weighted down with chains.

"What are those chains about you, Marley?" Scrooge asks.

"I forged these chains link by link when I walked the earth," Marley replied. "You, Ebeneezer, don't feel the weight of your own chains about you."

In the light of Cayce's philosophy, Marley had become "earthbound" by his attachments to materiality. His entire life and focus were on material wealth. When he died or made the transition, Marley found himself "weighted" by his own creations: greed, material gain, and wealth. These were his own heart's desire—Cayce called that situation "earth-earthy."

Marley's self-created hell was one of regret and lost opportunity. All material things pass away, and Marley was in a void, caught in the realization that he had built nothing spiritual he could take with him at death. Scrooge, trying to make Marley feel better, says: "But, Marley, you were always a good man of business."

Marley replies, "Business! Mankind was my business!" His hell was realizing that he did not practice love and kindness, but instead chose money and ruthless business practices. In his after-death state, he was haunted by what he did not do. Marley was unable to move in the material world, but also unable to leave it. A hell indeed! Yet he came to Scrooge to help Scrooge out of his own predicament. Even though he was chained, Marley was seeking to help Scrooge. If Dickens were to have written an epilogue to his classic tale, I imagine it would state that Marley was set free when Scrooge went through his own transformation on Christmas Day.

As Cayce often said in the readings, heaven really is not a place we go to at all; rather, we *grow* to heaven leaning on the arm of someone we have helped.

It was such a simple concept. No wonder people returned from near-death experiences profoundly changed. They saw that love was the only thing that mattered. People had reported seeing the panorama of their lives, and they witnessed all the striving for social acceptance, material gain, wealth, and power, and it meant nothing in the presence of this divine Light. Love, most people reported, is the only thing that lives on. All events of our lives will be based and judged on our ability to love. Everything else is secondary.

My fears of death were ebbing, and their passage felt like the dawn of the first day of spring after a long, cold winter, leaving me peaceful, new, and alive. I began to sense that eternity was now, in the present, and not some place where we go forever. If the Cayce readings were true, we are forever. It's only a matter of realizing it and living it. Now.

———

Hugh Lynn Cayce was a wonderful mentor to me. He led me to understand so much in such a brief amount of time. Yet, all during the time I counseled with him, I had no idea he was suffering from terminal cancer. I think of the responsibilities he had—the chairman of the board for A.R.E. and a worldwide author and lecturer. The weight of the world must have been heavy on his shoulders, yet he took time out for a twenty-year-old kid who needed assurance that death is not the end; all the while facing the inevitability of his own imminent death.

———

I was transferred to a six-week school in San Diego in June 1982. It was there that I received word from a friend about Hugh Lynn's own transition on July 4, 1982. *Independence Day.* After reading my friend's letter, I sat down for a period of meditation to send Hugh Lynn light upon the path of his new world. For the first time in my life, I felt that death was not the end, and I prayed a prayer of thanks for Hugh Lynn's guidance. If Edgar Cayce was right—that we grow to heaven helping others—I felt assured that Hugh Lynn had indeed gone to a heavenly home.

I never forgot what Hugh Lynn said to me, "You've got a lot of work to do here." I didn't understand at the time; I only hoped that eventually I might be able to help someone as Hugh Lynn had helped me. My wish was to be granted some years later. It represented one of the greatest gifts I have ever received. It also was one of the greatest challenges I have ever faced.

9

◆

*T*he remaining years in the navy were rich with experiences from my inner and outer travels. I continued daily meditation and developed the awareness that I was never alone. It was more a knowing than a belief, as if the act of meditation connected my awareness with a greater awareness or consciousness. As a result, I believed I was being guided and directed in my life's experiences. I imagined there were unseen protectors enveloping me like a cocoon, invisible companions along life's way. It was a comfort for me to believe in the Cayce readings' philosophy that each of us is guided by unseen and benevolent forces. Believing this, I was never far from the spiritual source that I made a personal part of my life and awareness. Consequently as my life changed from shore duty to life at sea aboard an aircraft carrier, I didn't agonize over the changes and adjustments. There was the sense that everything was happening according to some plan. I had been guided to Norfolk, Virginia; this was evident to me during and after I met Hugh Lynn.

For the first time I felt the comforting absence of fear and in its place was a sense of adventure and expectancy. This was the reason I joined the navy: to travel to the places I at one time had only dreamed of seeing.

Someone once said that life is a blank canvas and we are the painters of our own lives upon it. If that is true, one experience during the time I was on a seven-month deployment in the Mediterranean is painted in the most brilliant hues upon that canvas.

We anchored off Haifa, Israel, during the Christmas holidays of 1984. I took a three-day tour to the Holy Land. As I walked through the ancient cities of Bethlehem, Nazareth, Bethany, and Jerusalem, I was filled with awe. I became a part of the heights and depths of biblical history, and the feeling was not foreign to me. In Jerusalem, I walked the Stations of the Cross in old Jerusalem, silently marveling at what a long and arduous journey it was to the hill of Golgotha. As I reached the top of that hill, I was overwhelmed by questions and then a revelation: My God, what were the Master's thoughts on the day of His crucifixion? Jesus not only faced His death, He carried His cross to it. And here was I, standing upon the hill where He left this world. I could almost hear His final dying words from the cross echoing all around me: "It is finished." He accepted His death as a willing sacrifice for a world He loved beyond His own material life, a world He loved even though it betrayed him.

The sun was setting on the hill of Jerusalem and our tour group was descending from Golgotha, but I remained for a time. There was something of meaning for my life, at age twenty-three, here. I couldn't place it, but it was very important. It was as near to me and yet as invisible as a wind.

Pain. Courage. Grace. Forgiveness. Faith. They were all here — they were all necessary. Yes, the Master Himself forgave His persecutors, willingly walked to His death, and became the symbol of all life only at the point of His death. Not merely acceptance of death, but an example of courage beyond the finest definition of the word. Did He have fear? Did He have nightmares and worries and fears of His own mortality? I believed He did. After all, He was human. If He did not face the challenges, fears, uncertainty, and loneliness that we all face, then I believe His death would have been meaningless.

Standing on the hill on that warm winter day in Jerusalem, I believed in my heart that death did not come easy even for the Son of Man. Before the pronouncement, "It is finished," (John 19:30) He endured the dark night of His own soul: "Father, if it be thy will, let this cup pass from me." (Matthew 26:39) And then, "My God, why hast thou forsaken me?" (Matthew 27:46) I knew as I stood on the ancient hill that there was fear before courage and acceptance. I was learning to understand life and to let go of my fear of losing it only after embracing and feeling the fear and uncertainty fully. Must fear die before faith is born? I had so many miles to go to understand.

These words came to me: "If you will know Me in the calm, you shall know Me—and I shall be with you—in the storm."

"I will," I said aloud to Him and Golgotha. "I will know You in the calm and the storm."

I watched the sun set over Jerusalem, still not wanting to move from the place where life had defied the shackles of death. "I will know You in the calm and the storm," I said again. Words of prayer fell from my lips. They were a plea, an affirmation, and a hope:

"Teach me to face my life without fear. Inspire me to face my death with courage even as You faced Your own. Be near me in my own dark night of my own soul. May the storm of that night pass quickly. May the dawn of the calm come early. Amen."

I stood in silent gratitude for my life's experiences that had led me to the day and the place where the greatest, most inspiring drama of all time had played itself out. My tears were not the tears of loss or sadness, but an expression of thanks that I was alive and worthy to stand in the same surroundings as the Master. Here I was, face to face with something familiar and vast and powerful, something that I was not separate from. I was standing on the hill that had inspired love and war and peace and dissension and hope.

As I descended the hill, I was reassured of what I knew in my heart and had always known: *All is well, my friend.*

"Thank you," I said to the hill, the sky, the dusk, the Master. "It is not enough to say, but thank you."

———

My other journeys paled in comparison to my Palestine experience, yet I visited and celebrated history. I stood among the ruins of Pompeii and looked at Mt. Vesuvius, wondering what were the last thoughts of the people of Pompeii before Vesuvius ended their earthly lives. I stood in the arena in Rome and could almost hear the screams of the early Christian martyrs. I walked through the Vatican and nearly worshiped the crowning glory of Michelangelo's work, the ceiling of the Sistine Chapel.

I meditated in the Chapel of Apparitions in Fatima, Portugal. I sat with people from all over the world who came to pay homage to a place where the mother of Jesus spoke to the children of innocence. Her message was not unlike her own Son's: "Be at peace . . . love one another . . . I am with

you." If there were fifty of us in that chapel from fifty na-
tions, it was mere illusion. In the common bond of silent
prayer, we were seekers of truth from different lands, but
we were one.

——

As I completed my travels abroad, I felt that the navy had
served its purpose for me. I decided to return to Morgan,
Indiana, for a year before making a decision about what I
would do next. Virginia was now home to me, but I needed
to return to my family and friends for a brief time to reflect
and write about my experiences. It was in many ways a sabbatical early in my life. I was only twenty-four, but the
experiences I had been through made me feel much older.
Seeing what I had seen and feeling what I had felt, I knew
my spirit was as ageless as the hill of Golgotha. This awareness made me feel warm and safe and guided. But above
all, I was humbled. The answers to the questions I had
sought were answered with more questions about life,
death, and God and my relation to it all. The beginning of
the wisdom I had gained was realizing how little I knew.

10

◆

I was one of the millions of Americans who were glued to their television sets in the latter days of July 1985. National and local news stations were scrambling to build news stories around the prepared statement of Dr. Michael Gottlieb, a Los Angeles physician:

"Mr. Hudson is being evaluated and treated for complications of Aquired Immune Deficiency Syndrome."

Rumors had been running rampant about film star Rock Hudson's failing health for months. To the majority of Americans, Acquired Immune Deficiency Syndrome (AIDS) was a new and frightening phenomenon. Since 1981, news reports on the mysterious killer-disease were scarcely reported except in states dramatically affected by the rising death tolls: California, New York, Florida, and Texas. Suddenly, the deadly syndrome that destroyed the body's immune system had a celebrity face.

Before the announcement of Rock Hudson's diagnosis of AIDS, the fatal disorder was an anonymous disease that claimed the lives of the faceless and the unknown. Little attention was given to AIDS because the majority of the victims were homosexual men and intravenous drug users. In 1982 the disease had initially been called G.R.I.D.—Gay-Related Immune Deficiency. With Gottlieb's announcement, AIDS suddenly was on the cover of every newspaper and magazine across the country. Just as suddenly, millions of dollars from the federal government were promised for research. Gay activist groups were outraged. They had been campaigning since 1980 to raise the public's awareness about AIDS with little success. Critics were vocal and caustic to the press, asking where the front-page news stories about AIDS had been before a matinee-idol fell victim to it.

The gay community was understandably frustrated: They were the hardest hit and had the largest numbers of AIDS-related deaths. AIDS had surfaced in the United States in 1979. By the end of July 1985, 6,079 Americans had died from AIDS-related complications and 12,069 had been diagnosed with the disease. Seventy-two percent of the cases were among homosexuals.

I had been hearing about AIDS since 1983, when I was overseas. One of the sailors aboard the U.S.S. *Eisenhower* was diagnosed with AIDS that year and was quickly flown to a hospital in Italy. He died a year after his departure from the ship.

It was a puzzling contrast for me to see how Europe and the United States were dealing with the developing epidemic. In France, experimental laboratories were set up almost immediately after the first AIDS cases were discovered. The French government released its research findings about AIDS at every opportunity. The Pasteur Institute in Paris had become the leading authority on AIDS. It seemed strange to me that in the United States, neither the government nor the media wanted to deal with the disease. Consequently, they kept the public-at-large uninformed about AIDS even in the light of medical evidence that the disease was communicable. However, a small but well-organized group of physicians, scientists, and researchers acknowledged the possibility that AIDS could become the worst health crisis since the Black Plague. This group, who had tracked the disease's inroads into the United States, became the bearers of dark prophecy, warning that the death toll from AIDS in America would be 200,000 in a decade if people were not educated and warned about the sexually transmitted disease.

I read the latest news articles about AIDS in an Indianapolis newspaper. After the announcement about Rock Hudson, there was a new and different story or angle appearing every day concerning the growing epidemic.

I was troubled by the fact that a fatal disease that had been and was spreading at an alarming rate had been under-reported because of social stigmas. I wondered about the people with AIDS. What did they go through? I understood that death from AIDS-related complications was particularly grisly. When the immune system was destroyed, innumerable viruses and infections rapidly spread throughout the body. Death was usually slow and painful. I couldn't imagine facing death from a terminal illness with the attendant emotional upheaval, and I couldn't grasp the added cruelty of a society that was indifferent to such tragedies.

I was horrified to hear fundamentalist ministers proclaim in newspapers and on television that AIDS was punishment for the sinful, the sign of the end times, and a deserved fate for the wicked. Such pronouncements took me back to my boyhood encounter with the fundamentalists and the minister's preoccupation with scaring the "hell" out of me. How could these self-professed messengers of God be so callous as to say that AIDS was a just punishment for anyone? I felt hopeless and helpless as I now read first-person accounts in some of the larger and more open-minded newspapers of people who had AIDS and who were ostracized from their communities, who became destitute, and were abandoned by friends and family. These people were like the biblical lepers, feared and hated in this era by some of the well-educated in America who responded through misinformation and panic. People began running scared without any factual basis. Conclusive evidence showed that AIDS was not spread by casual contact.

I remembered my experience during my visit in Palestine and the feelings of love and acceptance. Even with the dark elements of my shadow side, my weaknesses, and my sins, that acceptance was real. When I stood on that hill of Golgotha, I experienced what until then I had only read about: unconditional love, the sense that the Creative Forces or God accepts us as we are, where we are. It was such a contrast to the anger, fear, and prejudice I was sensing in Middle America's response to the growing AIDS epidemic.

The challenge for me was to face the AIDS issue with love and forgiveness, a challenge in view of my anger about humanity's inhumanity to itself. The Master's words would serve as a daily affirmation for me in the days ahead: "Forgive them, for they know not what they do." (Luke 23:34)

In my own corner of the world in the Midwest, particularly Indiana, the public was dealing with the early days of the AIDS epidemic with not only predictable fear and misconceptions, but with displays by many of open prejudice against people with AIDS. In my hometown of Morgan, Indiana, for example, the editor of the town's newspaper carried reports about the "perverts" who had contracted AIDS, displaying the word "perverts" in the headlines when referring to people infected with the AIDS virus.

I became caught up in following a story about a young boy with AIDS that challenged the most forgiving hearts. I was witnessing a clear picture of just how fear can affect a community of people.

One of the first children who contracted AIDS lived in Kokomo, Indiana, less than twenty miles from my home. The child's name was Ryan White. At age thirteen, he was suffering from the early stages of the disease, but was still well enough to be in school. Ryan was a hemophiliac and had contracted AIDS through a contaminated blood-clotting product called Factor.

Ryan White and his mother Jeanne were dealing not only with the complications of AIDS, they also were dealing with the treatment they received from the townspeople of Kokomo. Because of Ryan, the state of Indiana created guidelines to determine when a person with AIDS was a risk to other individuals. Indiana's health commissioner had stated that Ryan could attend school as long as he was physically well enough. However, the day after the commissioner had made his announcement, the board of Ryan's school voted to keep Ryan out. After word got out about his illness, Ryan and his family were enduring a seemingly endless nightmare of persecution from residents in his hometown. A lawsuit was filed by Ryan's mother against the school board so that Ryan could return to school. Ryan's attorney argued that the school was discriminating against a handicapped child. The judge wouldn't make a decision until Ryan's attorney presented proof that the school was discriminating against Ryan. Until the case was settled, Ryan could not go back to school. In response to the White family's suit, fifty teachers from Ryan's school publicly announced they would refuse to teach him.

The insensitivity of some sectors of the Kokoko community left me feeling angry and frustrated. Kokomo, Indiana, is comprised of well-educated, upper middle-class citizens. I wasn't able to comprehend the effects of fear and ignorance until I read the continuing newspaper reports on the plight of Ryan White. He was a child; yet he was being treated like a dangerous criminal. Death threats were made to Ryan and his family. When the White family attended church services, they were asked to sit in either the front or rear pew so that the congregation would know where Ryan was at all times. He and his family had attended that church all during Ryan's life. His grandmother had been active there for years. After the services, parents quickly ushered the children far away from Ryan. Eventually, the minister informed the White family they were not welcome at the church. The hysteria grew, and soon Ryan and his family were alone. None of Ryan's friends were allowed to visit him, and the townspeople turned their backs on a dying little boy.

Mothers canvassed the town, petitioning to keep Ryan out of school. Students began taunting Ryan when they saw him and his sister in public. Parents began to speak out to the media.

"We've got to protect our children from AIDS," one mother said.

A constant stream of physicians was attempting to counter the growing unease concerning AIDS by telling the media that it was indeed safe for Ryan to be in and around other children. Precautions needed to be taken only if he was vomiting or bleeding. Yet, fear-crazed Kokomo threatened to remove their children from school if Ryan attended. The school offered to send a tutor to Ryan's home, but no teacher would take the job.

News stories of Ryan's plight were publicized throughout the country. He was quickly becoming the symbol of an ostracized segment of society: people with AIDS or what social workers called "PWAs". It wasn't long before stories about other people afflicted with the fatal disease began to surface. Interviewers talked to young men who had been abandoned by their families—literally thrown out of their homes because of their AIDS diagnosis. One man was beaten to death in San Francisco when a group of thugs learned that the man had AIDS. The stories went on and on.

Amid the controversy, I was calm in my anger. I cultivated it, however, quietly—like a nightshade garden. I had a sense of indignation and outrage, but in the center of it was a calmness of perspective. The epidemic had awakened something within me that I couldn't define. I meditated and prayed for guidance and waited and read on and on about the epidemic. I had had the same sense of imminence when I found the Cayce information. It was as if the higher aspect of my soul was beckoning: "Listen closely. This is important." I felt as if I were waiting for instructions.

I knew innately that the people of Kokomo were reacting from fear, but it was a dangerous, all-consuming fear. Their fear of getting AIDS made them forget they were dealing with a child who was facing a death sentence. Didn't they realize he was just a child? They were not seeing Ryan White the person, but were seeing a disease instead. The days passed, and I watched the pathetic face of Ryan White on the news tell people he wasn't dangerous, he wasn't a threat, he just wanted to go to school. Meanwhile, the court battle raged on for nearly nine months—Ryan White was still out of school and he was getting sicker. The White family couldn't go into a restaurant without people getting up and leaving. When Ryan and his mother Jeanne went into a restaurant in Indianapolis, the owner refused to bring them glasses of water. Instead, the waitress brought two cans of soda. After they finished their dinner, the owner ordered the waitress to throw out their dishes. This event was not done discreetly after Ryan and his mother left the restaurant—it was done in front of them. It got worse long before it got better.

Rumors and false accusations were made about Ryan and his family.

One of the kids from Western Junior High telephoned Ryan at home and accused him of spitting on vegetables at the local supermarket. Ryan vehemently denied the accusation.

"My cousin saw you," the boy said. "My cousin doesn't lie. He says you sneezed on them, too." As it is always the darkest just before the dawn, an amazing thing happened: Hollywood came to the rescue. The AIDS epidemic was no stranger to the entertainment industry, and they—unlike Kokomo, Indiana—embraced their own who had fallen ill with AIDS. Many celebrities used their fame to advantage. Elizabeth Taylor, Michael Jackson, Donald Trump, Meryl Streep, and a host of other major celebrities were in communication with Ryan and his family, openly offering support. Soon, Ryan's face appeared in magazines with other celebrities promoting awareness and education about AIDS.

AIDS had a child's face now—and that child vowed as long as he lived he would dedicate his life to helping people become aware of the facts and myths about AIDS. I was moved beyond belief—and that movement was the "something" I had been waiting for. I knew if I decided to become a volunteer for people afflicted with AIDS, there would be controversy—I didn't know how my parents would react or my friends. In the end, it didn't matter—people were being abandoned by families; they were being fired from their jobs, and they were dying.

11

$\blacklozenge$

Ryan White's story was a major reason I decided to get involved with the terminally ill. The work of Dr. Elisabeth Kübler-Ross was another factor in my decision. Through the years I had read books written by this remarkable physician. She created hospice care centers and instructed lay people as well as medical practitioners how to lovingly deal with the terminally ill. I initially came to read of her work to help alleviate my own fears of death.

Before Dr. Kübler-Ross began her unique life's work, it seemed to me in retrospect that the terminally ill didn't have a voice. Physicians are taught to cure and heal—but what happens when there is a patient who is never going to get well? Even in the early part of this century, cancer was treated like a contagious illness. Those so afflicted were often hidden in back bedrooms and treated like shameful secrets. Dr. Kübler-Ross, through her books, lectures, and workshops, taught millions of people around the world— including me—that death is a natural part of life and it should be treated as such. Her message was direct: the living have quite a bit to learn about life from the dying. She became the voice, the light, and the hope in the lives of the dying. For this, she became a great inspiration for me.

During the time of Ryan White's ordeal, I reread her book *On Death and Dying* and felt a call to service. Ryan White's story had moved me very deeply. The idea of becoming a part of a support system for people with AIDS felt like a natural part of my journey. My earlier sense of "something important is coming" came to fruition when I read the closing of Dr. Kübler-Ross's book. I knew then it was time:

> "Those who have the strength and the love to sit with a dying patient in the *silence that goes beyond words* will know that this moment is neither frightening nor painful, but a peaceful cessation of the functioning of the body. Watching a peaceful death of a human being reminds us of a falling star; one of the million lights in a vast sky that flares up for a brief moment only to disappear into the endless night forever. To be a therapist to a dying patient makes us aware of the uniqueness of each individual in this vast sea of humanity. It makes us aware of our finiteness, our limited life span. Few of us live beyond our threescore and ten years and yet in that brief time most of us create and live a unique biography and weave ourselves into the fabric of human history."

I was ready to touch that falling star. I was ready to enter the silence that indeed goes beyond words. In working with the dying, the experience would perhaps give me a chance to be of help to those nearing what Edgar Cayce called the transition and the passage through "God's other door." I would come face to face with my quest to fully understand the nature of my life and my eventual death and dying. I had dedicated several years to study and introspection about my life and its meaning. The time had come to take that work and make it practical. The years, the travel, the books, the hours with Hugh Lynn, and the journey through the dark shadows of fear and uncertainty—all were my training and initiation.

After reading that final passage in Dr. Kübler-Ross's book, I picked up the telephone and dialed the Indianapolis AIDS Education Outreach Hotline. I signed up for a two-day training seminar. I had read in the newspaper that the newly formed AIDS support group in Indianapolis needed volunteers to help care for persons with AIDS. It was a major event in my life to make such a quick decision. But I believed my experiences up to that point decided it for me. The majority of my life had been spent questioning, searching, and wondering about the meaning of our brief interlude on this earth. My introduction to religion from the minister, the LSD experience, my mother's near-death encounter, the Cayce information—all of these were leading somewhere. Something "clicked" when I considered working with the dying. Intuitively, there was a sense that this experience would be of great importance to the rest of my life. It was more something I had to do rather than something I thought would be charitable or would enable me to do something worthwhile for society. I suppose in many ways it was a selfish motive—needing to be near those who were approaching death so that I might know, in some way, that their passage was certainly not the end of their lives. Perhaps my helping them to face their own fears of passage would enable me to face my own.

I knew that I would be met by resistance in my endeavors, if Kokomo was any indication. But in my mind and heart there was no choice. Ryan White was one boy with a great dilemma weighing heavily on his young shoulders: he was facing his eventual death with absolutely no support or encouragement except from his immediate family. How many others were being treated as outcasts? How many were there that the media didn't talk about? In the moments that I thought of Ryan White, I heard the unheard voices; their cry was for someone to please stop treating them *like* a disease and see that they were people *with* a disease. They were asking to be set free from the bondage of injustice, prejudice, and fear.

———

The two-day training seminar at Methodist Hospital in Indianapolis was intense. Social workers, psychologists, and nurses, as well as people with AIDS, spoke about their experiences with the disease.

"You are in for the hardest, most brutal experience of your lives," a social worker told us. "But it can also be one of the most rewarding. I'm not going to tell you this is easy— all of you are here to help people who are not only dying, but many of them have been abandoned by their husbands, wives, friends, and parents. My hat is off to you for being here today. We desperately need each and every one of you." I appreciated her being candid and honest with us. She also gave us a warning:

"It's not just the families that are abandoning people with AIDS. Plenty of doctors and nurses are refusing to treat people with AIDS. You're going to have to be stronger than you ever imagined."

She gave us instructions on how to report nurses and physicians who refused to treat AIDS patients in hospitals. "It's a violation of the Hippocratic Oath for them not to help these people. Sometimes they have to be reminded of that—in writing." She smiled and I imagined she had written up her share of medical personnel. I wondered how she came to be a part of the support system for PWAs. I decided to talk with her during the break.

Her name was Jeanette and she had been involved with the epidemic ever since her mother-in-law had contracted AIDS through a blood transfusion in 1982.

"They treated her like a leper in the hospital," she said. So, I wasn't the only one who saw the analogy to lepers. "The nurses would leave her food trays outside her door." Tears welled up in her eyes. "Do you know what the worse part of this is? This behavior isn't uncommon. I'm sorry to say, but it may be 1985 and there's more media attention about AIDS, but ignorance is rampant, and a lot of people with AIDS are not being treated well." Someone called her to the telephone. "Nice to meet you, Rob. I'm glad you're here." Before I had a chance to say likewise, she was gone.

A news team had arrived to film a segment for the evening news. I hadn't told my family I was taking part in the workshop and wondered what they would think if they saw me on the news. Even so, I didn't hide from the cameras as they panned across the thirty or so participants in the seminar.

A nurse stepped up the podium after the break.

"I need to get something clear to all of you right away. There are a lot of rumors—most of them untrue—about the way AIDS is contracted. I want to first tell you the ways you cannot get infected: shaking hands, kissing, breathing the same air as a person with AIDS, eating or drinking after an AIDS patient. There is no evidence to support that AIDS can be contracted through casual contact. Not one piece of evidence.

"If we could contract AIDS like the common cold," she said, "I guarantee you we would all be in this hospital right now as patients instead of caregivers."

In my heart I had known this all along. The last thing I

had worried about when I decided to get involved was becoming infected. Granted, it is a very real concern—but
something within me knew that AIDS was difficult to contract.

"AIDS is a sexually transmitted disease. It is also transmitted through intravenous drug use by contaminated
needles, blood, and blood products—transfusions." The
nurse outlined how to take precautions in the presence of a
patient's bodily fluids.

"It's common sense to put on rubber gloves when you're
cleaning up a person with AIDS, especially if they vomit or
have diarrhea. But to set your minds at ease, there is no reported cases of AIDS among family members or support
people who cared for a person with AIDS." She emphasized
this last sentence and looked over at the TV film crew.

"If you put nothing else on the 6:00 news, for God's sake
put that last statement in! Jesus, I've had a hard time with
that!" We laughed, but I could see her very real frustration in
trying to get the facts out to the public.

During the question-and-answer session, a number of perti-
nent issues came up. "I've seen news programs in which
doctors and nurses are wearing masks and rubber gloves
while attending a person with AIDS. Is that necessary?"

"It most certainly is," the nurse said. "But for reasons you
may not have thought of. Basically it's to protect the person
with AIDS. If you have a cold or flu, contrary to popular belief, a person with AIDS is more susceptible to get your cold
or flu than you are at risk for getting AIDS from them. Remember, we're dealing with people whose immune systems
are barely functioning, if at all. Your summer cold could land
a person with AIDS in the hospital. Do put on the mask and
gloves if you're not well. I can't emphasize enough the importance of monitoring your own health. If you're healthy,
there's no reason to use gloves even if you're giving the patient a massage, a bath, or what have you.

"Another question?"

"What kinds of diseases do people with AIDS get?" someone behind me asked.

"I was going to cover that later this afternoon, but in brief—people with AIDS are susceptible to a host of infections and diseases. Remember that no one dies from AIDS; it's the opportunistic infections that kill them. AIDS destroys the body's ability to fight infection. Primarily, people usually contract what's called PCP—*Pneumocystis carinii pneumonia*. The PCP bug is in the air, in this room, right now. But our bodies have built up the ability to fight it off easily. People with AIDS are extremely susceptible to it. There is also a strange cancer they contract—Kaposi's sarcoma. Usually it manifests as large purplish-brown lesions on the skin. Some people are extremely disfigured by the lesions. It's worse when it attacks the internal organs. Kaposi's lesions can cause internal bleeding. If they're in the throat, they can close off the air passages. Toxoplasmosis is a very dangerous opportunistic infection. It causes brain abscesses and spinal meningitis. It's contracted from having pets—cats, birds, especially.

"A terminally ill AIDS patient will frequently die of malnutrition. They can no longer keep food down, and they gradually waste away. They can also get severe colon infections which can lead to untreatable diarrhea. The body eventually dehydrates itself, and the patient dies."

This was a nightmare. My God! What these people go through! All I knew before I went to the seminar was that people got AIDS and eventually died. I had no idea such horrendous diseases played a role. My head was beginning to ache.

A woman in the back of the room spoke up. "I heard that a nurse was infected from taking care of an AIDS patient." It was the news reporter. The nurse was very thoughtful in her response.

"There have been a number of cases reported in which medical people have been infected with the AIDS virus on the job. Yes, a nurse was infected—but it was not through any form of casual contact or as a result of caring for an AIDS patient. She was carrying AIDS-tainted blood samples. The nurse unfortunately tripped going through the lab door and fell on the samples, breaking the tubes. The glass from the broken samples penetrated her skin. Needless to say, a substantial amount of contaminated blood entered her bloodstream. She is now testing positive for the AIDS virus.

"In another case, a physician was performing surgery on a person with AIDS. He sliced his finger with the scalpel. He is also testing positive for the AIDS virus." The nurse surveyed the room.

"Please be aware of the fact that in these cases AIDS was contracted from contaminated bodily fluids to the bloodstream. There is nothing casual about any of these cases. If you are bleeding and you come into contact with the blood of a person with AIDS, the chances are very high that you will contract AIDS. However, I may be somewhat of a rare case, but a couple of years ago I accidentally stuck myself with an AIDS-contaminated needle. I was drawing blood. I get my blood tested every six months. I'm negative." The room buzzed with hushed conversation.

"That's what I'm trying to say here—AIDS is very, very difficult to contract under casual circumstances. As a nurse, I've taken care of scores of people with AIDS, in every sort of medical procedure you could think of. I'm healthy."

———

We went through a number of small-group workshops and counseling sessions with the psychologists. We were evaluated to ensure that we would be capable support people for the terminally ill. On the second day of the seminar they led us through a kind of guided meditation. After we were brought into a relaxed state, the leader quietly said: "You have just been told you have nine months to live. How do you react? Let yourself feel this deeply—you have been given nine months to live. When you feel ready, open your eyes and begin writing."

It was a form of hypnosis, and I realized I was in a state of deep receptivity. When he said, "You have been told you have nine months to live," I felt the reality of it. Immediately I found myself in tears, as did others surrounding me. I opened my eyes and began to write in an emotional fury. I was not self-conscious because of my tears, as I was among an understanding group of people; most of them were in tears as well. I wrote that I wanted to do everything today—not to put off anything. I wanted to live to the fullest; and whether it be pain or joy, let me feel it fully. I was anxious and angry and resigned. There was so little time! God, please let me finish what I came to do. These were the thoughts and feelings. It wasn't until I neared the end of my essay that I realized I had been in a hypnotic state. I truly experienced what it had been like to receive a terminal diagnosis. It became one of the most important aspects of the training seminar: to be able to fully identify and empathize with a dying person. If I could not put myself in his or her shoes, then I would not be an asset in that person's final months or years.

The most touching aspect of the seminar, which reaffirmed my desire to go ahead with this work, was a testimonial of a person with AIDS. He walked very slowly to the podium, each step looked extremely painful for him. The nurse offered him a chair.

"No. I want to stand for this. I'll sit if I get too tired. Thanks, Rebecca."

I was shocked by his appearance. I could tell he was close to my age, twenty-three to twenty-five years old; but the ravages of AIDS made him look much older. He was gaunt and very pale. For the first time, I was face to face with someone with AIDS. Large purple lesions covered his arms and neck. He was so thin I wondered how he had strength to move at all. Before he began speaking, he held onto the podium and lowered his head, obviously in pain and very ill. The nurse got up to assist him. "No, really, I'm fine—just give me a minute." Worry was written all over the nurse's face as she sat back down.

"My name is Danny. Rebecca asked me if I was up to speaking with you. It may not look like it, but I am up for it." He smiled wanly, and I could see premature age lines etched in his face. God, he could have been sixty years old.

"First of all, I've got to tell you that if it wasn't for Rebecca," he pointed out the nurse who had helped him to the podium, "I would not be standing here today. She has been my support person. My friend. My world. Thanks, Becky. As all of you probably know, I have AIDS. I've been sick since 1984."

He paused and tried to take a deep breath. "I'm a little out of breath. I just got out of the hospital from *Pneumocystis carinii pneumonia*—my third bout. I'm real weak because of the antibiotics. They're trying to fight off CMV, a vicious little bug that can cause meningitis or can cause me to go blind. I'm telling you these things so you'll know what happens to people with AIDS. I'm lucky, really. Some people get ten to fifteen different infections that are life threatening. I only have five or six. That's some light in the dark, eh?"

I looked at the people surrounding me. Some people had haunted, shocked expressions on their faces; some didn't meet Danny's gaze. A woman sitting next to me was shaking her head, searching for a tissue in her purse. "Dear God," she whispered to herself, "I have a son his age."

"When people at my job found out I had AIDS, I was fired and lost my insurance. I had to give up my apartment and move back home with my folks. When they found out I had AIDS, they made me move, saying I'd give it to the rest of the family."

"God forgive them," the woman next to me said.

"My father hasn't spoken to me since. It's been hard. But I've learned that your true family doesn't have anything to do with blood relations. My biological family turned their backs on me. Rebecca and all my friends in the support group are my family now. They've helped me through the anger, the pain, the hospitals, all the crap that goes along with this God-awful disease." He paused again to gather his strength.

"Each one of you who decides to become part of this program will become family to someone with AIDS as well. Maybe the person you will get assigned to will have a supportive family. I can only hope so. If not, please prepare yourself to become 'the family.'

"All of you are here for different reasons. Maybe you have a friend or a lover who has AIDS. It doesn't matter, really, why you're here. The important thing is that you are here. People need help. But I want to tell you that none of this is easy—for the person with AIDS or the support person or the family. There's a lot of anger here from all sides. I was very, very angry after I was diagnosed with AIDS. I felt cheated out of life. It was bad enough that I was sick, but the way society and my family were treating me—that added a whole other dark element to it. Rebecca has been a godsend to me—and I know I've been a royal pain in the ass at times.

"So please understand if the person you're assigned to doesn't seem to appreciate your efforts, or is angry, or doesn't want to talk. It's not you. A lot of us are in our twenties—many of us were just beginning our lives. It goes beyond frustration. So, yeah, you'll encounter the anger. When it all comes down to it, I'm trying to face all of this with some shred of dignity. That's a difficult task when you're in the hospital and they treat you like a specimen instead of a person. It's hard to keep your dignity when people look at you like a freak and are scared of you. It's hard when you lose everything. If you think I'm a rare case or story, you're wrong. There are hundreds, if not thousands, of Ryan Whites out there. Society is scared of AIDS—they won't educate themselves about the disease, they just want to be scared and that makes them dangerous. I tried and tried and tried to educate my family to let them know I'm not dangerous, I'm not a threat, I'm not contagious. They wouldn't listen. In the end, my parents didn't see their son any more; all they saw was AIDS." Danny wiped a tear from his eye. I wondered if this is what the lepers in the Bible went through.

"So, yes, people are turning their own children out onto the streets. It's not unusual. It's wrong—but it's not unusual. That's why we need people like you.

"I've listened to the TV ministers say that AIDS is a curse from God and punishment for the wicked and all that. Well, the God I believe in would never do this to me. For whatever reason I got AIDS, I'm going to make the best of it. I refuse to look at things like I'm 'dying of AIDS'; I'm doing a hell of a lot more than that—I'm living with AIDS and doing it the best way I can. And well, if the fundamentalists are right, that this is a punishment from God—then in my opinion God is a lunatic that needs to be stopped."

Maybe it was the tension and the sadness and the myriad of emotions floating around in that room—but the room roared with laughter and applause. I couldn't have agreed with Danny more. The God I know had better things to do than visit a plague on humanity. Even Danny was laughing, surprised by his own humor and eloquence.

"Thank you all for coming—and thanks for listening."

The woman who was fishing for a tissue stood up unannounced and spoke aloud what she had whispered earlier. "I have a son your age, Danny." Her voice began to falter. "And I'm so sorry—God, I don't know what else to say, I'm so sorry. I'm coming up to give you a hug." She was crying as she approached Danny. She went to him as a mother would embrace a son. Danny broke down and cried as well. "If you were my son," the woman said, "I'd be so proud of you! The courage you have to face all of this. I don't know you, but I love you."

Others came up to the stage. It looked like a picture of a family reunion. Strangers—but no longer strangers—embracing a weary human being who was facing the greatest challenge of his life. I thought that if it is true that we come to the earth for soul growth and development, as I believed we did, then Danny had graduated.

Everyone sat down. Danny remained at the podium. "I want to leave you with something. Let me say that I've learned more about life and living and loving in my dying than I realized in my healthiest days. You know what? It's the little things that matter to me now. Friends, the group, Rebecca, making it through another day. If you'll learn nothing else from people like me, you'll learn how much one day can mean. If it took AIDS to bring me to the realization of how precious time really is, then maybe it isn't a curse at all—maybe this is what I came to learn. Thank you all for being here."

As Rebecca went up to help him to his seat, people gave him a standing ovation. Danny may have been on the brink of exhaustion and barely able to stand during his talk, but the strength of his spirit shone through like a beacon. I joined the room in the ovation.

12

◆

I was contemplative, tired, and emotionally drained during the thirty-minute commute to Morgan from the final session of the training seminar in Indianapolis. Yet I never felt clearer about my decision to be a part of helping people with AIDS. However, the closing comments made by the nurse haunted me as I drove westward on Interstate 70:

"These two days are not enough to prepare you for what you will be facing in the days to come. As a nurse for more than fifteen years, I thought I'd seen it all. AIDS is the most devastating disease I've ever seen. The virus is some sort of monster. The ravages upon the patient are monstrous, physically as well as emotionally. You'll have to be very, very strong. This has only been a crash course in caring for people with AIDS. Actually, even if we had two months, that wouldn't be enough time to prepare you for what you are about to face. But we, as well as the people with AIDS, need you. And we'll be here to help you in any way we can."

She was like a warrior attempting to prepare and lead us to meet an enemy—"the monster" as she called it—face to face.

Like many people venturing off into this unknown territory, I hoped I would be strong enough to face what lay ahead. Not for myself, but for the person to whom I would be assigned. Above all else, I wanted to be a capable support person.

People who were professional hospice careworkers had also attended the seminar. An instructor told us that since AIDS was a relatively new disease—the first cases not surfacing until 1980—there was still much to learn about this mysterious illness in the eyes of the medical community as well as in society. Cancer hospice workers were there because cancer didn't have the damaging sociological issues attached to it that AIDS did. Part of our training was to learn how to deal with the prejudice and ignorance that went with AIDS. George Whitmore summed up the distinction between the two diseases in his 1988 book, *Someone Was Here—Profiles in the AIDS Epidemic* (Plume), which I read later:

"AIDS isn't like cancer. Cancer is frightening, but respectable."

The nurse was candid with us in stating that science was far from knowing all there was to know about AIDS. "You're all going to be learning about AIDS right along with the rest of medical professionals. We're all still learning about the implications and complications of this disease."

AIDS was complicated and unpredictable because science, medicine, and sociology knew so little about the disease in 1985—six years into what AIDS statisticians were calling "a future holocaust."

Medically, a new infection was being discovered regularly

among AIDS patients and registered with the Centers for
Disease Control in Atlanta. There didn't seem to be an end
to the ailments that could afflict a person whose immune
system had collapsed. The scientists were scrambling just
to track and chronicle the opportunistic infections. Medical research became another issue. Lobbying groups for the
CDC and the National Institute of Health were practically
begging for research money from a federal government
which had been and was dragging its feet on dealing with
the epidemic since it began. It was taking much too long to
acquire the funds needed to research AIDS.

Sociologically, there was the specter of fear with which
the public was reacting to AIDS. Ryan White's dilemma in
Kokomo had painted a graphic picture of how irrational and
panic-stricken the public could become in dealing with a
person afflicted with AIDS. In 1985, there was the continuing misconception in the Midwest that AIDS was only
affecting the gay community and I.V. drug addicts. This
made AIDS education more difficult. At that time, stories of
cases of AIDS among the heterosexual community and
among children were seldom reported.

It was all overwhelming to me. I was motivated to be involved, but I felt incredulous and bewildered at the same
time. All of the issues surrounding AIDS seemed so vast and
complicated.

Even though I was becoming educated about the medical, social, and political issues of the disease, I often had to
remind myself that I was getting involved to be a caregiver,
not to be a politician or a sociologist. So many issues surrounding AIDS awakened a sense of indignation in me. I
needed to remember my ideal was to be a help to someone
with AIDS. My emotional nature could be a hindrance if I
wasn't careful: I was carrying around a great deal of anger
and frustration at how the AIDS crisis was being handled.
Even though the treatment of Ryan White was one of the

factors which brought me to be involved in this work, it could also sidetrack me into getting into the politics of the AIDS crisis. There was another factor which added to my already volatile temperament over the issue: the pronouncements of some sectors of the fundamentalist religious groups. Their openly proclaiming that AIDS was punishment for the sinful added fuel to my already raging fire within. I envisioned showing them a picture of a child with AIDS and asking them to explain to me the "wickedness" for which God was punishing that child.

I could see that more disciplined meditation would have to be a mainstay for me during these times. I needed to find that calm within, for there could be many volatile storms on the horizon.

Above and beyond my personal insecurities and uncertainties, my job would be to create the most loving and supporting atmosphere possible for a person with AIDS. "Support person" were the key words in my role.

I thought about the portion of the seminar that dealt with the five stages a dying person goes through in order to cope with a terminal illness. Kübler-Ross had outlined those steps in *On Death and Dying*. The dying were not the only ones to go through the denial and isolation, anger, bargaining, depression, and eventual acceptance of their passage. The family, close friends, and even the caregivers experienced those phases as well. An instructor told us we all experience one or another of them in the stages of our life: the end of relationship, a change of career, the loss of a loved one. Any major transition in life is accompanied by the journey from denial to acceptance.

Always in the back of my mind was the persistent questioning. Was I strong enough to do this? Do you really intend to do this? It was a voice I was familiar with; it was the voice that wanted me to run away from the things that were painful. The answer to that voice was enough to silence it: *Yes, I*

intend to do this. I have to. I need to. The inner conviction
was strong and undeniable. In retrospect, I can see that this
was to become a life-transformative event. I believe there
are pinnacles of opportunity that happen in our lives, and
we have the choice to take advantage of them or pass them
by. I could have passed this opportunity by, but there was
an echo in the deeper part of my soul or spirit that said, *This
is important.* No reasons given. It felt a part of why I was
here on the earth at this time. The sense or feeling was that
strong. My intuition told me that the experience of encoun-
tering death and dying was going to make the life of the
person I was assigned to and my own life more meaningful.
Furthermore, the deeper spiritual part of myself that had
led me through the unusual experiences of my life had a
deeper and more meaningful reasoning behind my endeavors: *You believe in the survival of the soul upon death. But
there are people facing great crises who aren't sure about that
at all. They need you. They need the reassurance that death is
just a passage, a journey.*

It was all the reasoning I needed.

———

Arthur Martin, the coordinator of the AIDS support volunteer service, had told us at the close of the seminar that
he would contact each of us when the Indianapolis AIDS
Task Force received word from a person with AIDS or the
individual's family, who needed assistance from a hospice
volunteer. The task force tried to pair up people in close vi-
cinities.

A couple of weeks after the training seminar, Arthur telephoned and spoke with my father, leaving a message for
me to call back. It was urgent. That was the entirety of the
message. When I received it, I knew that Arthur was going
to assign me to someone.

My folks are not people who intrude into others' affairs—

even their own children's. Arthur's telephone call, however, puzzled my father. It was rare in Morgan, Indiana, to receive an "urgent" phone call unless someone had died. They were concerned.

I took the message from my father, ignoring his and my mother's concerned expressions. I had not yet told them about attending the seminar. As I dialed Arthur's telephone number out of earshot of my parents, an inner voice was insistent: *You're going to have to tell them—soon.*

"Hello?"

"Hello, Arthur, this is Rob Grant."

"Oh, hi, thanks for calling back so soon. The reason I said it was urgent was because there is a young man named David who needs help. He lives in your hometown. David stays with his mother and grandmother. His mother is divorced and works most of the time. His grandmother can't get around so well. Arthritis. They called and asked if someone could help them out."

"Yeah, sure," I said. "Did you say they live here in Morgan?" I hadn't heard of any cases of AIDS in my hometown. But given the controversy surrounding AIDS at the time, it didn't surprise me.

"David does live in your hometown," he repeated.

"What's his last name?" I asked.

When Arthur told me David's last name, I felt as though someone had knocked the wind out of me. I had known David while I was in high school seven years earlier. He had graduated in 1978, a year before I did. We had been in several theater productions. We had never become close friends, but we always got along well during the plays.

My God, David has AIDS?

"Rob, are you still there?"

"Yeah, Arthur—I'm sorry. I was just a little shocked. I know David from my high school days."

"Wow, Rob. I'm sorry. Were you close?"

"We had a lot of fun during the school plays, but we didn't hang out much."

"Listen, Rob, I need to tell you this—David is not in good shape at all. He just got out of the hospital last week. He's got chronic-active hepatitis, tuberculosis of the bone marrow, very close to pneumonia. He has difficulty keeping food down and he has a bacterial infection that's causing persistent diarrhea. He's lost a lot of weight. He's also having trouble walking."

David was having trouble *walking?* The image of the David I knew in high school was not at all the person Arthur was depicting to me now. David had been a champion swimmer, a star athlete. He also danced for all the high school musicals.

" . . . he's been diagnosed since 1984."

While Arthur had been talking, my mind was calling up images of David from high school.

"Arthur, I'm sorry, I'm still reeling from the news—I wasn't listening. What did you say about him being diagnosed since 1984?"

"He had been sick for a while before the AIDS diagnosis, but most of the medical testing was done there in Morgan. They didn't know what was wrong with him."

Morgan was not advanced when it came to medical care. I could only imagine the way the small-town mentality of the physicians-in-charge viewed David when they found out he had AIDS.

"What can I do, Arthur?"

"I've called his mother and told her about you. Her name is Marianne and she's handling all of this wonderfully well under the circumstances. She was so appreciative that someone would be coming to help out and just spend time with David. She said he'd been so lonely. I wish all parents who had children with AIDS were as receptive and caring as she is."

I had worried during the seminar that I might have some serious confrontations or problems with the family of the person I was assigned to. I was relieved. A supportive family meant a big and positive difference.

Arthur gave me David's telephone number and then he reemphasized David's deteriorated condition. I felt he was trying to prepare me mentally to see David.

"He may be in the final stages of AIDS, Rob, I just don't know. According to my files, I *do* know that David is in a much more advanced condition than any other case we currently have on our client list. I'm telling you this because you knew him before he got sick."

Deteriorated condition. Much more advanced. Final stages. The words seemed so final, so *ending.*

Well, of course, they are—what did you expect when you got involved with this, Rob? You're dealing with people who are very ill—they have AIDS.

I felt a sort of displacement—like a kid who had joined the army, thinking it was the right thing to do at the time, then coming face to face with the boot-camp drill sergeant who's yelling: "What did you expect, kid? This is the army, not summer camp! There's work to be done here!" It was a psychic command of sorts for me to get a grip on the reality of what I was involved in.

I had learned much about AIDS and the people it was affecting, and I had learned that a global crisis was at hand. But I had grasped these things at an intellectual level. I was feeling the distance between intellectual reasoning and the mind-heart feeling of the situation, the *reality* of the situation. The difference was experience. I had done well with the book learning. Now I had begun the real education of experiencing. I marveled at the distance between the two.

Arthur and I were talking about a human being. Not an idea. Not a concept. A living, human being who, more than likely, was facing death at a very early age.

Something clicked. I felt some psychic movement from thinking to feeling. I was beginning to experience the impact of all this. Maybe it was because suddenly AIDS had a face—not of a stranger, but of someone I had known. My reasoning mind had taken a side trip and left me with my raw feelings. A powerful surge of emotions ran through me that brought me face to face with a sense of selfishness.

What had I been thinking this was all about? I had been dealing—perhaps for years—with some abstract idea about what I thought life and death and dying meant? Trying to find answers to *my* search. There was a young man in my hometown who probably never dreamed of facing these issues—especially at age twenty-five. David probably never wanted to deal with anything other than athletics and the arts and living. Now he didn't have a choice.

With these thoughts came anger at myself, a frustration that I had perhaps missed the most valuable point of it all. A paraphrased passage from the Cayce readings came to mind: All knowledge is to be used for the assistance of others.

Over the years, I had been so busy trying to figure things out, looking at the mechanics of the universe to pursue something illusive and supposedly spiritual that would help me gain . . . help me gain what? And for whom? For me, of course, only for me. How presumptuous and selfish! Of importance here was life—mine and someone else's; a human being who was dying. I should have been focused and thinking about the person I would be helping.

13

◆

I told my parents about David before I met him or his family. It was the afternoon of Arthur's call. The situation was an uncomfortable moment for me. I didn't initiate the conversation; Dad was concerned about the urgency of the telephone message.

"Who is Arthur?" he asked. My mother, father, and I were in the middle of dinner.

I was tense and defensive. We had never discussed AIDS. At this point, I was vague in my answer to my father. I decided that now was not the time to discuss it.

"Arthur assigns people to work with the terminally ill," I said, not looking up from my plate. "I went to a two-day training seminar to learn hospice care. I'm going to volunteer for them a few days a week."

My mother was startled.

"What?" Dad asked, surprised but not disagreeable.

"I knew I shouldn't have said anything about this," I replied, feeling more defensive than ever. "You wouldn't understand."

Mom sensed my frustration. "I didn't mean to sound as if I didn't *approve* or understand—it just caught me off guard. Rob, it takes special people to do that kind of work. I think it's wonderful you're going to help out. I guess when I sounded surprised, I was thinking out loud—that I couldn't do that kind of work. If you can handle it, you are very special."

Her reassurance put my defenses at rest. "Thanks, Mom. I hope I can. It's hard to explain, but I just feel as if I need to do this." Even though the tension was easing around the dinner table, I still was not being completely honest with either of my parents. I decided to provide a few more details.

"Arthur called to tell me that there's someone in Morgan who needs help. He's dying. I said I'd spend a few evenings a week helping out. His name is David, and I knew him from high school."

There was an awkward silence. Then Dad broke the silence by asking the question I knew was coming:

"What's the matter with him?"

"He has cancer," I lied.

———

Not much more was said about the situation that day. I felt guilty for not telling my parents the truth about David's condition. Part of me rationalized that I was easing them into the idea by first telling them I was working with someone who was terminally ill. Then I would tell them David had AIDS. The other part of me said I was a coward. I was simply fearful of the unknown: I had no idea how my parents would react to my working with people with AIDS.

I telephoned David the following afternoon. The AIDS support group was meeting in Indianapolis that evening. I didn't know if David was up to attending the meeting, but I thought it would be a great way to get to know him.

Our conversation was light and easy. He recalled our days in theater in high school. I gently brought up the subject of his health.

"How are you feeling, David?"

"I feel as if I've been sick forever. I'm doing better. My temperature is only 101 degrees today. Yesterday it was 103. I have good days and bad days."

"Are you up for company?" I asked.

"Please," he replied. "I would love it. I don't get much company these days. And I want you to meet my mom and grandma. They've been just great to me." David's voice sounded vibrant and healthy.

"There's an AIDS support group meeting in Indianapolis this evening at seven o'clock, David. Do you feel up to attending?"

"It sounds great. I'll see how I'm feeling later on. But I would like for you at least to come over for a while anyway."

"Great," I said.

David said that he sometimes starts his days out feeling fine, but feels worse as the day goes on. He said he didn't know how he was going to be feeling from hour to hour.

He gave me directions to his house. Before I left, I looked through my junior-year high school yearbook, when David was a senior. There was a swim-team photograph of him doing a backward flip off a high diving board. In one of the group photographs, David had the appearance of the all-American athlete—blond, well-built, and with a winning smile. I remembered he was about my height—5'8" or 5'9". I leafed through the yearbook to the theater production photos. There was David as one of the dancers in "Hello, Dolly!"

He's having trouble walking now. Arthur's words haunted me. I couldn't fathom what David must be going through—from a star athlete to the depths of this disease. A chill ran through me.

As I drove to David's house, it was unusually bright and sunny for an Indiana winter afternoon. December is normally gray and overcast. I parked the car in front of the one-story, red-brick house on the corner of Mason Street. I could see the Christmas tree through the living room curtains. It looked to be a cheerful home.

David's mother, Marianne, opened the door for me.

"Hi. I'm Marianne. Please come in." I introduced myself and her smile put me at ease. She looked to be in her mid-to-late forties. She had dark hair with attractive gray highlights. She had what I had always called "smiling eyes." Yet I could see the lines on her face in that smile. It betrayed the stress and strain she must be enduring with her dying son.

She introduced me to her mother, Lillian. "I'm so glad that you could come," Lillian said. Lillian, who looked to be in her late seventies or early eighties, reminded me of my great-grandmother. Seeing her smile the way she did made me feel at home. I could sense the love in their house and that they were a very close family.

"David said he knew you from high school," Marianne said, leading me to the living room. "You both used to be in the plays and musicals."

"We had a great time," I said. The living room walls were decorated with family portraits as well as original watercolors and pastels. I wondered who had painted such vivid landscapes and abstracts. From the portraits I could see that Marianne had a large family—at least five children. I recognized James, one of David's older brothers. He had graduated with my brother John.

"David is lying down right now," Marianne said. "He really wants to go to the support group meeting tonight, but he wants to be rested. I'll get him up in a few minutes. Tell me about yourself."

The story of how I had arrived in their home came easily. I had imagined there would naturally be some awkwardness in meeting David's family. There was nothing awkward at all. I found myself in the company of an extended family I had not yet met in this lifetime. It felt like home to me. I remembered Richard Bach having said that strangers are friends and family we've not yet met. They welcomed me not as a stranger, but as a friend.

I talked about Ryan White and the struggle he and his family had been enduring since the residents of Kokomo found out he had AIDS. Marianne then spoke freely about her son having AIDS.

"Back in 1983, David was having all kinds of physical problems. No one knew what was wrong with him. He had all kinds of tests run. He had been diagnosed with hepatitis, but that didn't account for his sudden weight loss. He lost thirty pounds within a month." She paused and looked toward her mother for a moment. I could see they were both reliving those uncertain days.

"Finally," Marianne said, "I asked our family doctor if he might have AIDS. I had read about it in some magazines. Dr. Johnson—he's our doctor here in Morgan—got real defensive. 'Why would you think that?' he asked me. I didn't want to tell him that I'd known David was gay for years and that he had spent a lot of time on the West Coast, where some of the first AIDS cases showed up."

"What did you tell him?" I asked.

"I told him it was 'mother's intuition' and asked him to run some tests—whatever tests needed to be done.

"And . . . and they ran the tests," she said. Her voice was starting to waver and I wanted to comfort her—but wasn't sure how. She reached for a tissue.

"I'm sorry, Marianne, I didn't mean to —"

"No," she interrupted, "I *need* to talk about this. I need to talk about this with somebody who understands. Don't be bothered by my tears. I cry off and on a lot these days." She half-heartedly laughed, wiping tears from her eyes and I wondered how she could laugh at all. Lillian sat beside her, and I could see a bond of closeness. She was telling Marianne it was all right to let it out.

I often think that stopping up emotions is to help not the person crying, but to save the person they're with from being uncomfortable. I had learned a long time ago that letting the emotions out is the *best* way to get to feeling better.

"They told me he had AIDS," Marianne said. "I don't even remember which doctor or nurse it was who gave me the news. I didn't hear anything else he told me. I just kept thinking, 'My God, my son is going to die—what am I going to do without him?' I didn't know much about AIDS, but what I had read left me feeling so low and depressed. David was getting sicker and sicker before my eyes. I couldn't— and can't—do anything to stop it."

Marianne looked into my eyes as if searching for answers, answers I wished I could give her. She looked at me a long time before she added: "I've seen the news reports on Ryan White, too. It's an abomination what that family has been through." Her face flashed with anger. "I've also seen where parents are abandoning their own children because they have AIDS.

"David is my son *first.* He *has* a fatal disease. He is not the disease. I cannot believe these people who are abandoning their children—their own *flesh and blood*—throwing them out into the street because they have AIDS. What mother— I ask you—what mother would disown her child because he was *dying?*"

I told her about Danny and the story he told of his family believing he would infect the rest of them. I found myself recounting the story with the same bewilderment Marianne had expressed.

"Excuse me for saying this, Rob, but that is so much bullshit. I've read so many things on AIDS. You can't catch it like a cold. I know how people get AIDS. We take precautions around here when David vomits or if he's bleeding. I *knew* in my heart we would be fine taking care of David at home. He's not a risk to anyone. I wouldn't have it any other way; David belongs with his family during this time."

Oh, if only the rest of the world felt that way! I thought.

The conversation lapsed, and it was one of those rare occasions when the silence is not uncomfortable—especially when meeting new people. We sat, lost in our own thoughts. I let the moment linger without speaking. I could feel a bond with these people. I felt a sense of belonging. Also there was a familiar sense of "presence" in the room, very similar to what I had felt in Palestine. Guardian spirits, perhaps? I had a deep sense that I had indeed been guided to this family.

"How are you both doing?" I broke the silence. "I can only imagine how difficult this has been on you." Lillian and Marianne looked at each other and smiled. Their expression reminded me of comrades who had been together through the battles, war, darkness—and who had come out amazed and happy to be alive.

"It's hard," Lillian said. "Marianne lost a son before David. Michael was only five years old when he died of lymphoma."

My God. Lymphoma was a cancer of the immune system. The symptoms are very similar to AIDS. *How in the world has she held up through this?* I wanted to reach out to her, but I remained still. She nodded her head as her mother spoke.

"It's hard because David looks so much like Michael. I just can't understand the way the Lord works sometimes."

I couldn't either.

"I don't think we're supposed to know, Mom," Marianne

said. "We're just supposed to go through it all and thank God for the strength we have to face it. Maybe one day it will make sense."

I decided to be candid with my beliefs. "I remember reading somewhere that at the end of our lives here on earth, we come to understand the nature of all things." I explained what people reported from near-death experiences, the panoramic view of every thought and deed experienced in one's life. I also spoke about the incredible, all-knowing, all-loving Light.

"People reported that in that state of consciousness everything made sense—all the questions and puzzling issues they had during their lives suddenly were understood with clarity. When these were revived, they didn't have that universal knowledge any more. It's as though we can't know the real truth behind all the circumstances while we're here—but only *after* the life is lived, then we understand. I've often thought that if we knew that the situations in life were merely learning experiences or lessons, then we wouldn't take them nearly as seriously."

"Sort of like knowing the answers to a final exam in school," Lillian said. "If we knew the answers ahead of time, I guess the test wouldn't show what we had learned."

"Well, I would certainly like to talk to whoever is giving me *my* final exam," a very loud, comical voice spoke from behind me. We all turned and there was David, leaning against the kitchen table, smiling at us. "Because I don't like the course—and I want my tuition refunded!"

While David was laughing at his own joke, Marianne got up to give him a hug. "I can always count on *you* for comic relief, David. How long have you been listening in?"

That's David? If he weighed more than 115 pounds I would have been surprised. As we looked at each other, I could see that David knew exactly what I was thinking: *Oh, he looks bad.*

"David, you remember Rob?" Marianne asked, introducing us.

I got up and moved toward him, carefully shaking his thin hand. "Hi, David. It's been years since I saw you."

"Don't tell me," he said with mock seriousness, "I never looked better, right?" I knew the humor was a defense mechanism.

"David is notorious for black comedy," Marianne said. "He jokes about everything."

David looked at me soberly. "Sometimes I feel that if I can laugh, even when I feel like screaming, I'll make it through another day." I nodded, saying nothing.

Looking at David, I could feel that there was a part of me that wanted to scream, even though I was smiling at his jokes. There was a "before-and-after" series of pictures running through my mind of the David I knew from school in 1978 and what was left of David standing in front of me now.

Oh, yes, they are right; this disease is a monster.

The only thing that had not changed in David's appearance over the years were his eyes—they were still sparkling and intensely blue. However, if I had passed David on the street earlier in the day, I would not have recognized him. AIDS had robbed him of youthful qualities. He looked like a man in his late fifties. I was shocked. Perhaps I wasn't as shocked at Danny's appearance because I hadn't seen him during the time he was physically well. However, David did not have the Kaposi's sarcoma lesions, nor did he look as emaciated as Danny.

"I do feel up to going to the group tonight," David said, almost shyly. "Will you take me?"

"My limousine awaits," I said, bowing toward the door. "Actually, it's a Chevette, but we can pretend."

"What, no chauffeur?" he asked.

"I gave him the night off."

"How good of you," he said in a British accent. I was glad

to see the old theatrical David.

Lillian and Marianne looked at each other with amused expressions. Something unspoken passed between them. Marianne then ran off a verbal checklist of medicines David needed to take with him and made sure he had his coat, scarf, and gloves. We said our good-bys, and I helped David to the door. From the way Marianne was fluttering about him, I suspected David hadn't been out of the house in a long time.

I held onto David's thin upper arm and back as Marianne opened the door for us. "My legs and feet are swollen," David said. "Edema. I have to walk slow."

"That's O.K.," I said. "I'll follow your pace."

It took a long time to make our way down the thirty-foot-long sidewalk. As I opened the passenger door of the Chevette, I helped him get situated. He was frustrated at how long it took him to get settled in the car.

"I'm a pain in the ass," he grumbled.

"No, you're not, David. You're doing fine."

"It's ridiculous how slow I move. Thanks for coming," he said. He looked at me as I got in the driver's seat and smiled.

"I'm glad to be here," I said. I was.

14

◆

*T*he AIDS support group meetings were held in Dr. Daniel Marcus's office in downtown Indianapolis every Monday evening. They had been held there for the last seven months, ever since Dan found out his brother had AIDS. Dan was an internal medicine specialist. He worked six days a week and kept his office open late on Mondays for the group. The meeting room was spacious and decorated in shades of teal and mauve. Comfortable couches and chairs were arranged in a circle. I recognized one or two of the people from the training seminar I had attended. I expected to see Danny there.

I practically carried David into the office. The five-block walk from the car to the medical building had exhausted him; we had to pause every half-block so that he could catch his breath. By the time we reached Dr. Marcus's office, David was breathing as if he had run a marathon. Having recently recovered from a respiratory infection, he was still suffering a shortness of breath.

I was thankful that the office was on the first floor. Dr. Marcus met us at the door, quickly introduced himself as Dan, and helped me get David to the couch in the meeting room. Some people were already there. They came over to us.

Again the thoughts: *What happened to the athlete?* I was close to a state of panic, my mind disjointed. *What happened to the dancer? What in the name of God is this thing that turns a healthy twenty-five-year-old into an old man?*

Fifteen minutes after we arrived, David's color was still ashen, his breathing patterns were erratic, and he was holding his stomach in pain. I was grateful to be surrounded by people. I didn't know what to do.

"Pills," David whispered, practically hyperventilating. His face was a grimace of pain. Dan knelt beside David holding a glass of water as I took a bottle of pills from his coat pocket. Marianne told me he might need them for pain. I read the label, "Take one or two tablets every three to four hours as needed for pain." *Dilaudid 2 mg.*

"How bad is it?" Dan asked. "Do you want to lie down for a while?"

David shook his head. I handed him two of the tiny orange pills. He took them immediately with a small sip of water. The eight or nine people around us were silent, vigilant. Arthur came in and knelt beside Dan. Some silent understanding passed between them, then Arthur sat beside David, rubbing his back. He saw that I was anxious and he smiled, saying everything was all right. Nothing seemed all right, but Arthur's smile reassured me.

He's used to situations like these. How in the world does anybody get used to this?

Dan was taking David's pulse. I put my hand on David's

shoulder to let him know that I was there. I didn't know what else to do.

"David," Dan said after a few moments, "are you sure you don't want to lie down for a while? I've got a nice comfortable couch in the other room."

David opened his eyes, finally beginning to breathe easier. "What?" he said, still whispering. "And miss all the fun? No thanks. I want to be with the group." He smiled despite the pain. A cramp seized him, doubling him over. I wondered aloud to David if his discomfort was from the hepatitis.

"It's my liver, yeah. It's been swelling. A lot of pressure. I need a new one." He laughed weakly.

"Attaboy!" one of the group members said. "Laugh when you feel like crying. It takes less effort." David nodded at the man, and they both smiled.

"I'm feeling better," David said, regaining his voice. "What an entrance, eh?" The crisis seemed to have passed. I put my arm around him. Everyone sat back, looking relieved.

"Danny went back into the hospital several days ago," Arthur said. He had had a convulsion and was being treated for cryptococcal meningitis, a brutal and often painful opportunistic infection that causes a host of complications, including brain abscesses.

Five people in the room had AIDS. Only with David and the man who had said "Attaboy!" was it obvious. The latter had Kaposi's sarcoma and was emaciated.

Arthur opened the group meeting by formally introducing David and me. Then all in the group introduced themselves and told a brief personal story of how they had come to be a part of the group.

I was surrounded by people who were grappling with an issue that most of the world avoided. It seemed unusual to me that the people in the group dealing with these matters were thirty years old or younger. Faced with the challenge of their lives, they related candid and poignant stories that touched my heart. I thought they were all so brave, even when they expressed their fear and uncertainty.

The people with AIDS spoke of the little things of everyday living that most of us take for granted: Having a good day. Being strong enough to go for a walk outside. Feeling well enough to have company. Eating a good meal and keeping it down. Living for another day. It was a sad twist that made them appreciate the best of life only when the things taken for granted are removed—things like health, family, a secure job, a lover or husband or wife. Many of the people in that room had lost all of that and more.

———

David had shared one of those little everyday things of life I so often overlooked as we were driving to the group meeting:

"Oh! Look at that sunset," he said, gazing out the passenger window. "It looks just like a painting, doesn't it?" He turned his face toward me—his eyes were childlike, filled with awe.

"It is beautiful," I said. It was dusk. The sun was setting over the rural hills of Indiana, pouring hues of red, yellow, and gold over the landscape. Taking in the sight, I felt a pang of guilt. David was viewing this as if it were the first sunset he'd ever seen. I felt the guilt plainly: Of the days and months and years I had passed the sunsets and sunrises in my life, how many times did I see the majesty and beauty of nature around me and just assumed it would be there tomorrow?

David was living and seeing, as Dr. Kübler-Ross had said, as if each day were his last—as if this sunset was the last he'd ever see. Perhaps, I thought, this is the gift that the terminally ill can teach the rest of humanity: What would the day look like to us if we knew it were our last on earth? It would look as perfect and as beautiful as David was seeing it.

In silence he turned his attention back to the outside world that had become foreign to him since his illness. AIDS had taken its toll upon him physically; he was weak and fragile. Yet there was a vibrant light in his eyes; life never looked more brilliant to me as I watched David's face gazing at that sunset.

David then did something he would do many times during the next six months. He read my mind.

"You'd think I've never seen a sunset before!" he exclaimed, coming out of his reverie. He looked away, embarrassed.

"I know it may seem silly to you. But I don't see this often. Since I've been sick, I've had a chance to think a lot about the things I've taken for granted. This means the world to me."

"It's not silly at all," I said. "You know, it's beginning to mean the world to me, too," I said. I cleared the clutter of thoughts from my mind and saw the brilliant sky through David's eyes. *God's canvas. The sky.* I was thankful for the reminder of the beauty of the moment.

David told me that he was a painter. He had been painting in oils and watercolors for years, ever since high school. I was never very adept at painting or drawing, but I had had a love affair with art since I was a teen-ager.

"Those paintings in your living room—they're yours?" I asked.

"Yeah," he replied shyly. "Do you like them?"

"You're not a painter, David. You're an artist."

———

"Attaboy's" name was John. He struck me as the mystic or spiritualist of the group. He was calm, serene, and almost intensely at peace as he talked of his life and AIDS. Physically, he was a mere shadow of his former healthy self. His eyes had a faraway look—almost as if he were daydreaming. I had seen it in Danny's eyes. I saw it in David's as well.

The purplish Kaposi's sarcoma lesions covered John's upper arms and his neck. Although John was visibly very sick, there was a calm about him. I didn't know it then, but I was gazing into the face of acceptance. He was not anxious or upset when he spoke.

"If they discover something new about AIDS," John said, "by my having it—if they find out something that will lead someone to feel better or even get well from this disease—if it helps even just one person—then all I have gone through will not be in vain. Nor will I have died in vain."

John's comments upset Jerry, a younger member of the group. He looked to be about twenty-two and very healthy. Jerry let out a sigh when John stopped speaking and wiped a tear from his eyes. "You're talking as if you're already dead," Jerry said. "Not everyone dies from AIDS."

John, with that same level of calm, smiled at Jerry. "You're right, Jerry. I still have some living here to do. I've learned to look at this life as a school—a place of learning. Look at me, Jerry."

Jerry had turned his attention to the floor when John began speaking, clenching his hands together nervously. He wasn't comfortable with John's philosophy. Finally, he looked up at John.

"We're all teachers," John said. "We're all students, too. How do I know that I didn't come in this life with this disease so people could learn? Yes, the doctors and nurses—the educated—they're learning from me. Maybe I'll provide some clue to the mystery of AIDS. Probably it will be after my death. When it's time for me to *graduate*, as I like to look at it, to another life, another world, then I'll go. I don't see death as the end. I'm not afraid, Jerry—really I'm not. I've lived a full life even in my thirty years."

I was close to tears, looking at this gaunt figure, weary, physically marred by a disease few understood, who somehow through a devastating illness had found himself at peace with what to me looked like a cruel fate. He had not only found peace in life, he had found purpose. This was at the heart of my search as long as I could remember: to find the purpose and the peace and to calm my inner restlessness. I was inspired by John, yet I had a long way to go before I would understand that peace.

"My having AIDS is giving people a chance to understand the incomprehensible," John added. "It's giving them an opportunity to learn."

This idea of the caregiver being the student and the patient the teacher brought back a perspective from the Cayce readings I had gleaned, but not understood until that moment. A reading was given for a family with a child who was born with a host of physical and mental problems that were not easily curable. The reading said that this child was an opportunity for the parents—the caregivers of a baby who was totally dependent upon them—to learn love, compassion, and care. There was more to this situation than pointless tragedy. The reading spoke to the parents at the *soul* level and said that they had chosen to be of service and to manifest love and compassion to this special soul. In showing the child love, the parents would learn love. Cayce stated that this seeming tragedy was of paramount importance to the spiritual and soul development of the parents as well as of the child. He said that the soul of the child was very "advanced" in the spiritual sense.

The family's being together was not necessarily for the child to become physically well from illness, but for that illness to provide an avenue for the parents to learn a divine aspect of helping.

I also remembered a movie I had seen some years before called *Resurrection.* In the movie, a woman had discovered that she had a gift of laying-on-of-hands healing after a near-death experience, and she began healing people. She wasn't able to heal all the people she touched, however. When a doctor asked her why she couldn't heal them all, she replied, "Doc, some people need their sicknesses so that other people can take care of them. Those people I can't heal." Illness, once again, was a teacher, an instructor for the people taking care of the sick.

Were the people with AIDS teachers in disguise? Beyond the findings in medicine, did the people with AIDS come to challenge and teach the world to learn compassion, tolerance, understanding, and love? That was indeed the theme of Kübler-Ross's powerful book, *AIDS—The Ultimate Challenge*. She saw people with AIDS as the teachers.

John's expression of acceptance of having AIDS did not make Jerry feel any better. If anything, it provoked him. In contrast to John's calm, here was Jerry, young, afraid, and angry. He had been diagnosed a few months before as being infected with HIV—Human Immunodeficiency Virus, the virus associated with AIDS. Looking at John must have been like looking into a mirror of the future—a possibility of what was to come. My anger was called into play when I looked at how young Jerry and John were. No one, in my mind, needed to go through such a brutal experience at such a young age. Part of me felt the serenity of John and another part the sense of injustice in Jerry.

"Well, I don't want to be a teacher," Jerry said. "I didn't come here to die a horrible death so somebody can take care of me. I'm not going to die. People survive. I just have to take care of myself."

"You're right," Arthur said, "not everyone does die from AIDS-related complications. There are people who are surviving and living healthy lives with AIDS." He paused and looked around the group. "It's not always terminal. But you've got to shift your attitude from 'I'm dying from AIDS' to 'I'm *living* with AIDS. And I'm living the best way I know how.'"

Arthur mentioned that in the coming weeks he was going to bring a videotape of Louise Hay, a woman who was working with people with AIDS using mental and spiritual tools such as creative visualization. Some of her clients had reportedly experienced a remission from AIDS and were getting well.

He asked the group why some people, given a prognosis of six months to live, died on the last day of those six months.

"Why do others live well beyond their prognosis? What's the difference?" Arthur asked.

"I think it's a matter of will," I said, speaking for the first time to the group. "Some people have a determined will to stay here and work through their illness and get well. Others have come, as John said, to teach others. Maybe that doesn't have anything to do with getting physically well." The group was silent. I continued. "I don't think it's a matter of 'denial' to refuse to accept a terminal prognosis. If you have something to go on for, to live for, I think any prognosis can be made to be of no effect."

Arthur agreed. He explained that the will to live is beyond living for a relationship, a job, or a career. He saw the will as a spiritual part of our nature.

"The will to live is beyond the physical," he said.

"But," John said, "I don't see the prospect of my dying as a matter of having a strong or weak will. I don't believe I am giving up. I am letting go. I feel I have almost completed what I came here to do. Letting go is *not* giving up." John had beaten his physician's prognosis: He had had full-blown AIDS for more than three years. Statistically, after the onset of the first opportunistic infection, a person with AIDS's life expectancy was from one year to twenty-four months.

David, feeling more comfortable now that the narcotics

were taking effect, said, "I'm afraid of dying. I'm afraid it will hurt. That's what I'm most afraid of. I see myself going downhill every day, and I hurt more every day. I don't want it to hurt."

Michael, a man in his early forties, talked of being with his companion when he died.

"When Bill finally died," he said, "I was with him. There was no struggle. He said three words to me right before he went." He paused, and it was clear he was reexperiencing Bill's death.

"What did he say?" David asked, almost whispering. I could see the fear in his eyes.

Michael wore the saddest smile I had ever seen.

"Bill said, 'Oh, yes. Deliverance.' Just those last three words, and he stopped breathing. He said them like you would say, 'Of course, this comes next—how could I have forgotten?'"

I was glad David had opened up about his fear of dying. I didn't know how to approach it. I watched David as Michael was speaking. I could see he was feeling somewhat relieved and hopeful, but still very cautious. It was evident that David hadn't discussed dying with anyone before. I was anxious to tell of the experiences of people who had had near-death encounters. Those accounts had helped me so much in my early years and alleviated a great deal of my fear.

Janie, the only woman in the group, spoke to David. "Living is the hard part—the physical suffering, the illnesses, and the pain. I think when it's time to let go, there's great relief."

I again remembered the Cayce reading which said that there are many more difficult things to go through in life than passing through "God's other door." Death was easy. The process of living up to that point of transition was difficult. Looking at David and the other people with AIDS, I was reminded of how difficult that process can be.

"Bill was definitely relieved," Michael added. "I saw it. I saw it in his eyes. I could almost feel his relief when he died. And why shouldn't it be that way? He left behind a body that was racked with pain and misery. The Bill I knew and loved went on to what I believe is heaven. After what he went through, there has got to be a heaven."

The energy of the group was rapidly changing. We didn't stay on one area or person very long. But the time spent with each was very intense. Time was a precious commodity here. A chance for us all to share in the horrors and trials and the fears and uncertainties. This group experience was very powerful.

"I was at the hospital all afternoon," Janie said. "I'm exhausted."

Janie had been with the support group since it started. She was assigned to a young woman who had been hospitalized with AIDS-related illnesses for the last several months. Mary was not able to walk any more; the combination of AIDS and being bedridden had atrophied her leg muscles. No physical therapist would help her. Mary had contracted AIDS through a blood transfusion in 1982.

"They treat her like a bug," Janie said. "I go by to see her every day, and three times last week I found her supper tray on the floor outside the door."

"Bastards," Jerry hissed. He was still staring at the floor, clenching his hands.

Janie got a tissue out of her purse and dabbed at her eyes. "Some of the nurses won't go near her. They don't give her the pain shots on time. I've yelled, screamed, and complained. I've written up a whole floor of nurses. The head nurse on the evening shift is the worst of them all. I'm sure she just tears up my complaints."

Although she was crying, Janie said these things with little emotion. She reported the series of horrendous events in a monotone. Janie had the same weary appearance and expression that Dan and Arthur had.

Jesus, this is a war, I thought, and lost my composure.

"The U.S. is in the seventh year of caring for people with AIDS," I said, not masking my rage and frustration. "AIDS patients are virtually helpless in hospitals. Why is this happening? What's wrong with these people? Can't we do something?"

Arthur said he had talked to the administrators of the hospital repeatedly about Mary's care. They assured him that food trays were always delivered to the patients, that the nursing staff was educated about AIDS, and that there must be some sort of mistake.

"They're lying," Janie said.

I felt indignation rise in me. That helpless girl was at the mercy of the hospital and an indifferent staff. If David ever encountered that kind of behavior, they would have me to deal with. I had discovered that I had a flaring temper in my teen-age years. It matured as I got older and became like a sharpened knife. No, they didn't want to encounter me on this issue.

During those months that Mary had been hospitalized, there had been repeated problems with her medical treatment. Since Arthur had already talked to members of the hospital staff, Dan said he would talk with the physician in charge of the infectious diseases ward. Arthur said he would rally a battalion of volunteers to monitor Mary's treatment at the hospital. For several days around the clock, Mary's care would be policed.

"If her care doesn't improve after that," Dan said, "I'll go to the newspapers or talk to the TV reporters. I just may do that anyway."

"I'm sorry about your friend," David said to Janie. "I hate the hospitals. I hate how people look at me and treat me."

"How do they look at you?" Arthur asked.

"Like they're scared of me. Like they don't want to go near me. You're the first group of people I've been around other than my family who aren't scared of me."

"They're not scared of *you*, David," Dan said. "They're ignorant and frightened about AIDS."

"Boy, aren't they! The few people in Morgan who know I have AIDS are also scared to be around me."

David told the group that shortly after he was diagnosed with AIDS, he went to exercise at the local Y.M.C.A. in Morgan.

"I went for a swim in the pool and did a few laps. A good friend of my mom's found out I had AIDS. She's very well-to-do and prominent in the school system in Morgan and all. When she talks, the town listens—E.F. Hutton-type thing." David was trying to make light of the situation.

"She found out I had AIDS. *Then* she found out I swam in the pool. Well, her daughter was taking swimming lessons at the Y.M.C.A. at the time."

"Oh, boy, I know what's coming," John said. "What did she do?"

"Panicked. In a big, big way. She made a lot of noise, demanding I be barred from the Y. Do you know what was done?" David didn't mask the sarcasm nor the hurt in his voice.

"They drained the pool," someone in the group said.

David nodded. "Not only did they drain it, they *scoured* it with bleach."

"We're lepers," John said simply. "That's what we're seen as." His face clouded for a moment. "People really are comical in their stupidity. You just have to laugh sometimes. It gets so ridiculous." John's voice began to break.

"What is it, John?" Arthur asked.

"I was just remembering when I was diagnosed with AIDS," he said. "Seems like a century ago. I was sick for so long, not knowing what was wrong. Then—boom: the diagnosis. I was so upset I called my parents. I didn't have a lover—I didn't have anyone I could really talk to. So I called Mom. She and I had never really been close, but I needed her, you know?"

The memory was painful for John. His serenity and calm were gone.

"I told her on the phone, 'Mom, I have AIDS.' She didn't say anything. She just sighed. I can still hear that *sigh*." John covered his face with his hands and cried. Arthur moved over beside him. "Let it out, John. You stuff your emotions. You need to let this out."

"My own *mother!*" he cried. "She'd never accept I was gay. She was a fundamentalist and told me it was 'an abomination.'" John spoke quickly, trying to rid himself of the memory and the hurt. There was sadness in his voice, but there was also relief. It was like a confession.

"I told her I never chose to be gay. I've just tried to make the best of it because I couldn't change. It was *me*.

"She told me this is what I deserved," John sobbed. "She said God was punishing me. Then she hung up the phone. She *hung up!*"

When he regained his voice, John finished by saying that when he went to visit his mother the following day, she had moved all of his possessions out into the front yard and locked the door.

"She hasn't talked to me since."

The stories of the group members' lives ran the gamut of all the stages I had read in Dr. Kübler-Ross's work—from denial to acceptance, from despair to hope. By the end of the evening, I felt as if I had known the group for years.

15

◆

*T*hat first evening at the group I saw an aspect of David that AIDS had not touched: his strength and compassion. When John lamented about his family and how they ostracized him, it was David who went to his emotional rescue. David asked John to call him anytime he wanted to talk, day or night.

"I don't know you very well," David said, "but I'm here for you. All of us are. I guess that's why they call it a 'support group.' "

We all voiced that we were in this together, but it was David to whom John gravitated. I think it was because they shared what, to the outside world, would look like a common weakness or illness. They were both physically in the same stages of AIDS. Their sickness brought them together, and that bond was powerful and meaningful. Each knew how the other felt; they were in each other's shoes. Although born of tragedy, John and David's budding friendship was bound with intense sharing of feeling and emotion. David reminded John that he, too, was ostracized—not from his family, but from the community in Morgan. He then told John something that touched me deeply.

"John, I used to be religious—in the church-going sense. There was something I learned from my years of church-going and reading the Bible. And it still means everything to me:

"Jesus was the king of the outcasts. He was the leader of the downtrodden, the scorned." David put a reassuring hand on John's shoulder.

"Jesus told us that when we are persecuted, remember that He was persecuted before us. Because of that He will be with us the whole way—through it all, 'even unto the end,' like He said."

John looked at David's smiling face. His eyes filled with tears, and he asked David if he really believed that. He asked not as a skeptic, but as someone who hoped desperately that there was *someone* on his side.

"Hell, yes, I believe it," David firmly replied.

"Dave, you have such a poetic way of putting things," John said, smiling.

John hugged David and held onto him like a long-lost brother come home. This time, it was David who said that everything was going to be O.K.

I was witnessing something vital and *real.* It was as if everything else in life paled in comparison to the almost fierce sense of love and harmony in that room. What Elisabeth Kübler-Ross had said is true—we are most vitally alive when facing and dealing with the imminence of death. It makes a meaningful moment all the more vital because time becomes so very short.

John and David in their moment epitomized the best and

worst of their lives. Their physical health ruined, they were deemed outcasts by society and family; they were dying. Yet, they had found each other in the very dark night of the soul, and from the depths of their beings they found strength to sustain the other.

David was right. Jesus *is* the king of the outcasts. If there were sides to be chosen, I had no doubt that He would keep company with David and John and the rest of us. We were the modern-day outcasts, the lepers. I was happy to be on the side of the outcasts.

———

It was shortly after my first AIDS support group meeting that I stopped watching the news. Little was being done to educate people about AIDS, church and state were divided on the moral and medical aspects of the disease, people continued to die from it. It made me too angry and frustrated. I thought I would eventually be of absolutely no worth to David if I was angry at the world's injustices. So I focused my time and energy on David. An interesting thing occurred. AIDS took a back seat in my thinking. David, as a person instead of a patient, became my focus as well as my friend. He was incredibly likable. He had a sharp, entertaining wit and took interest in everything around him.

"When you have everything taken away from you," he said on one occasion, "the only thing you really have left is a sense of humor. And if you don't have that, you lose your mind as well." David reminded me of the character Hawkeye from the movie *M*A*S*H*. Laughing at the horrors of the war merely to get through it with some sanity. He also made me recall what Edgar Cayce said about humor: to see the ridiculous side of *every* situation. David could do just that, and I admired him the more for it.

He gave me a new perspective on life as well, seeing the world with the eyes of an artist and always observing the interesting and the beautiful; things that I at one time over-looked. He relished old Bette Davis movies and would act out parts of the films. David was, after all, still an actor. He had a zest for storytelling and told me of his fast-track life on the West Coast, where he worked briefly as a model. David loved music and he still sang beautifully.

Although he was afraid of dying, he didn't feel cheated out of life. "If I die tomorrow," he said, "I can say I lived a full life." Indeed he had. After high school, David studied art for a year at Indiana University. Creatively restless, he decided he had had enough of art and went to Florida for what he called "a rowdy sabbatical." After a time in Ft. Lauderdale, he headed for the West Coast and joined the marines.

"Every gray hair I have on my head," Marianne said, "I attribute to David. His adventures worried me sick." David loved to rehash his past, but didn't want to look at photographs of himself from those days. It was too painful for him to see such a change. Yet he came to accept the burden of his deteriorating health and strived to do as much as he creatively could.

He continued his painting and occasionally wrote very moving poetry. He loved to play the piano. It was amazing to me because he kept busy even though he was feeling at his worst. I knew for myself that when I got a fever of 100 degrees, I was miserable. I didn't feel motivated to do more than turn on the television. David's fevers were always raging. He was in chronic pain from the tuberculosis and the hepatitis. He regularly battled respiratory infections and was always dangerously close to pneumonia. His coughing would wrack him to exhaustion. His once athletic and graceful body had become his enemy. But that intangible magic that made up David's soul would not give in nor give up. His spirit was bound and determined to be as creative as possible and express itself artistically even in moments of the body's greatest pain. His fortitude and long-suffering awed me.

I began to understand that although David was dying, some part of him was vitally alive. I loved to hear him play the piano. He would play completely improvisational pieces—and no two songs sounded alike. Listening to him, I felt I was in the presence of some divine gift. Although his body was wasting away, his spirit became more vibrant, more *visibly* expressed. He was nearing "home" in a spiritual sense. Perhaps it was like the flame of a candle that burns brightest just before it burns out.

My evolvement from being David's "social worker" to his friend came gradually and easily. It was a time of great vulnerability for me. How do you get acquainted with someone and then have to let him or her go? David was dying. I knew that. I think that's what made the time I spent with him so special. Kübler-Ross was right when she wrote that we are most vitally alive in the presence of death. We realize the preciousness of the moment. How wonderful the "now" is when it's all we have. This made it difficult for me as well. It was as though I were waiting for some macabre alarm clock to go off and suddenly David would be gone.

I began to spend more and more time in the evenings with him and Marianne and Lillian. I became part of Marianne's and Lillian's daily lives as well as David's. Those days were, like the nurse had stated at the training seminar, the most rewarding and the most heart-wrenching of my life.

I noticed that David was eating less and less each time I came for dinner. Sometimes he couldn't keep anything on his stomach except milkshakes and vitamin supplement drinks. Marianne would meticulously prepare foods she thought he could digest. It became a frustrating challenge for her. David would eat dinner or lunch. Fifteen minutes later, he would vomit. After these episodes, Marianne and I would help him up and take him to his room.

"I'm sorry, Mom," he said. "I tried to keep it down." We

would both shush David, telling him it wasn't his fault—he was sick. The anxiety on his face was clear to me. *If I can't eat, I'll die.*

One evening after we got David settled into his room, Marianne broke down as soon as his door was closed. It was rare for her to express her emotions. She had reached her breaking point, and in many ways I was relieved. She desperately needed to let out the grief she felt for her son. She was sobbing, and I took her into my arms.

"Dear God, what am I going to do?" she cried, and I just held her. "He hasn't kept any food on his stomach in three days! I don't think I can take it! Rob, how can I *help my son*?" It was a desperate plea. I held her tightly and cried with her.

"Please, won't somebody tell me! I'm his mother and I can't make it better—I can't make *him* better!" Her torment was excruciating. Day by day she was watching her son wither away, powerless to stop it.

"Every day," she sobbed, "every day I think, 'Oh, this time he'll be able to eat and it will stay down.' And he never does! He *never* does!"

"Marianne," I said firmly, not trying to stop her tears, but attempting to calm her, "it's not your fault. It's the AIDS. David can't keep food down because his liver is swollen; it's pressing against his stomach. It's too hard for much food to pass. Rather than passing, it comes up."

"When he vomits, I feel as if I've failed him. Do you understand?" It was a dilemma without solution or relief. David couldn't eat. I was powerless to help except to hold her and share her tears.

Again she pleaded, "Dear God, how can I help my son?"

———

There were long stretches in which David seemed to survive on minimal food. Then he would have days and weeks when his appetite was ravenous and his food would stay down. His condition was unpredictable.

I began to look into alternative health treatments that might help David stabilize, help him keep food down, be more comfortable, and in less pain. Always in the back of my mind was that *something might work—something in the Cayce readings has got to help David.* Marianne's faith never wavered; she held fast to the glimmer of hope, even though David was going downhill rapidly. We both wanted to believe in miracles.

I wrote to a supplier of Edgar Cayce remedies and requested they send me castor oil and wool flannel. Castor oil had become something of a miracle-worker for a host of different ailments during Cayce's lifetime. Cayce prescribed it a number of times in his psychic readings. It was processed from the Palma Christi plant (meaning "Palm of Christ"), and legend told that the plant was blessed by Jesus and contained healing properties.

From what I had seen in the readings, it certainly contained something that was indeed very healing. The readings recommended "castor oil packs" for numerous people. It was simple to prepare. Just heat the oil in a pan, and saturate a piece of wool flannel. To help David's hepatitis as well as his digestion, the flannel pack would be placed over his liver, a sheet of plastic covering it, then a heating pad placed on top of that. The pack was left on for an hour or more. It could be put on a number of different areas of the body for various ailments. The castor oil would be readily absorbed into the body through the skin, no matter where the pack was placed.

Sixty years before "transdermal patches" were developed by science to administer medicine through the skin, Cayce prescribed such treatments. People had written letters to him and to the A.R.E. in subsequent years reporting relief with castor oil packs from gall bladder problems, sprains and bruises, and hepatitis.

David was anxious to try it, hoping for relief from the abdominal pain and pressure. I hoped the castor oil packs would help. Within a week, the company mailed the castor oil and wool flannel, and I went to David's house. His family was open to anything that would help him at least feel better. An evening of castor oil packs eventually became a daily ritual in his household. They helped reduce his abdominal pressure from the hepatitis, and he was able to keep food down.

The first evening I brought the castor oil, I had no idea how David's system would react. I could only hope for the best.

"I keep expecting that he'll be able to keep his food down," Marianne said. Her eyes were large and frightened. "I pray for it. Do you think this will help?"

As we were heating the castor oil on the stove, I told her of instances in the Cayce readings in which people reported a lot of good from castor oil packs.

I went into his room and turned on the lamp beside his bed. He didn't stir.

"He hasn't been sleeping well at night," Marianne said. "His fever seems to go up at night and he's so restless. He had a bad day today. I finally gave him a sedative a few hours ago."

When David didn't sleep, neither did Marianne. The lack of sleep was showing in the dark circles under her eyes. I encouraged her to try to rest. According to Arthur, David would need more attention and assistance as time went on. Even though he was having serious medical complications as a result of the AIDS, none of them were life threatening at the moment.

I unbottoned his shirt and placed the castor oil pack over his abdomen. The outline of his liver was prominent on his thin frame. Marianne sighed as she looked at her sleeping son. Near David's lower abdomen were two hard lumps, the size of walnuts. Marianne said she didn't know what they were. I placed the flannel over his liver on his right side and over the two protruding lumps, plugged in the heating pad, and set it for medium-high. I wrapped a piece of plastic over the flannel, added the heating pad, and placed a towel over the whole pack. Still, David didn't stir; his breathing was shallow but even.

I turned out the light, and Marianne motioned for us to go into the kitchen. We sat down to have a beer. We enjoyed the quietude of the house.

A calm befell the home whenever David slept. A good night's rest was a rarity. He was prone to night sweats. The sheets and blankets would be soaked and have to be changed in the middle of the night. Diarrhea often kept him up as well. The fevers gave him bizarre dreams and night-mares. I was grateful that tonight he was sleeping peacefully.

Marianne, too, was relieved that David was resting. She kept her feelings of helplessness over his condition hidden most of the time. When he was up and about, she made it a point to always be optimistic; she talked only of things light and hopeful. She was painfully self-conscious about any-thing that might upset him as he had a tendency to fly off into a rage for no apparent reason. David was normally good-natured and gentle. But when he was feeling particu-larly ill or lonely, he would vent his anger on Marianne or Lillian. Marianne was always patient with him, but firm. On one occasion he flew into a rage because he couldn't keep his food down, and he took it out on Marianne.

"David, I'm sorry you're sick," she said. "But it's your con-dition, not my cooking." She never yelled at him, but she would lovingly and humorously put him in his place. Kübler-Ross had written in her books that some people who were terminally ill *never* got beyond their anger.

Marianne realized that when David did get upset over insignificant issues, he was really frustrated with having

AIDS. However, maintaining a positive environment for
him took its toll on her. She often smiled when she felt like
screaming. She would joke with him to keep his spirits up.
Her inner strength never ceased to amaze me. She faced the
days of David's illness with great courage. Yet she could not
hide the pain in her eyes. When I asked her how she found
the strength to carry on, her answer was simple:

"God gives me the ability to cope. I'm lucky to have my
mother with me, and all my kids and I are very close."

In the Midwest in 1986, there were no groups to help the
parents of AIDS-infected children. Marianne's support system consisted of the church, Lillian, several of her children,
and me. I caught on early that we were not to discuss the
severity of David's condition in front of him. If David wanted
to talk about his condition, it was discussed. It was important to Marianne to keep their lives as normal as possible so
that David would not feel as if he were being a burden.

"All of this wears on me," she said. "Sometimes I don't feel
as though I can take it. But I can't—I won't—let David know
these things. He's got enough to deal with." How lucky David
was! After the horror stories I had heard about abandoning
families, Marianne was a godsend. I told her so. Her response was appreciative, but sharp:

"I'm doing what any decent mother would do. May God
forgive the others." Marianne was helpful in teaching me
the importance of forgiveness.

"Those people are to be pitied, not hated," she said. "God
knows, it really is an effort for me not to get angry.

"And I don't give a damn if people are afraid of AIDS!
David is still a *person.*" Marianne was justifiably angry.

"Let's say just for the moment that you could catch it like
a cold," she said. "So what? David is my son. He always will
be, no matter what. Jesus said a lot when He told His
apostles, 'Greater love hath no man than to lay down his life
for his friends.' I believe that. Yes, I would die for my chil-

dren if that's what it takes. I thought all mothers would, but I'm wrong."

I thought of John's mother hanging up the phone, that final click in his ear.

"Yes," she added, "I forgive them and feel sorry for them. If they really understood or knew what they were doing, they wouldn't do it. I believe that, really, with all my heart."

Suddenly an image of Jesus arose in my mind. *Forgive them, Father, for they know not what they do.* The understanding of those words bloomed in my mind like a flower. It was a beginning for me of letting go the feelings of rage and injustice.

"Cheers!" she said, raising her beer in a toast. "I'm finding this helps me a lot these days."

"I'll drink to that," I said, laughing. Marianne chuckled and drank. She looked exhausted. She had a full-time job with a health spa, teaching swimming. Lillian was home with David during the day. I would come over in the early evenings and sit with David and Lillian while Marianne was still at work.

The months prior to my meeting David and his family, I had been involved with a local theater group, putting on plays in the evenings. I had just finished a production when I had attended the AIDS support seminar. I didn't miss the theater. My evenings and weekends with David, Marianne, and Lillian made me feel as if I'd always been a part of the family.

Marianne and I sat in silence for a time, drinking our beer. "David is a very special soul," Marianne said after a few minutes. "I'm not saying that because I'm his mother. I mean—he's—well, sometimes it's scary. It's not just his music or art. Come here, I want to show you something."

I followed her into David's room. He was still soundly sleeping. She turned the light on in his bathroom. What I saw was an exotic garden. I felt that I'd stepped into a greenhouse. Plants and flowers were in hanging pots, vines crawling up the woodwork. Everything was blooming.

Why are these flowers blooming? It's mid-January.

A chill ran through me as she knelt down and pointed to a flowerbox underneath the sink. David had built, quite intricately, a square box, six to eight inches deep inside the compartment under the sink. Petunias, impatiens, and other spring flowers were in bloom.

"David loves plants and flowers," Marianne said. "He's always had a knack for growing anything. He planted these just a couple of weeks ago." She was smiling, but startled at the same time. There was not nearly enough light in that room for flowers to flourish as these were. I looked up and saw a tiny window high on the wall, next to the shower stall.

It was eerie. It was fifteen degrees outside. The overcast Indiana winters made all the plants in our home go into a sort of hibernation; their growth slowed down.

"These are flourishing!" I said, awestruck.

"That's David," Marianne said. "But—what's really strange," she paused, choosing her words carefully, "as David has gotten worse, physically, his plants and flowers grow quicker. And these are *blooming.*"

Petunias. Blooming? How?

Marianne said she felt that it was a sign. A sign from God that, as difficult as all this is, David is going to be taken care of. I felt as if I were seeing something divine, some form of spiritual compensation for his tortured physical condition.

"David having AIDS is the worst nightmare I've ever had. But this little thing with the plants. It's almost as if something is saying 'everything is all right.'" Tears welled into her eyes as she looked at the indoor garden.

"Mom?" David was awake. Marianne and I must have looked pretty strange kneeling in his bathroom. She quickly brushed away a tear, not wanting him to see her upset.

We left the bathroom and came over to David. We turned

on the light; his face was flushed and red. When I felt his forehead, it was amazingly cool. *His fever was down.*

I sat beside him, still awed by the phenomenon of his mid-winter blooming flowers and plants.

"This is hot—but it feels good," David said, pointing to the castor oil pack. "I don't feel so much pressure in my stomach."

Marianne put her hand on David's forehead. She smiled at me, looking hopeful. "His fever is down." I said a silent prayer of thanks.

"I was showing Rob your flowers," she said.

"What in the world are you giving those plants, David?" I asked. "Steroids?"

"Nothing special. I just miss the spring and summer so much. I had some seeds from last year. Mom got me the soil, and I built the box and planted them. I wished for them to grow. I prayed for them to grow. I thought that if I can see the spring flowers, winter will pass quickly."

"David," I said, "there's not enough light for them to grow in that bathroom."

"They just like me, I guess," he said, grinning. "'The Lord moves in mysterious ways,' " he pronounced solemnly. Then he and Marianne started laughing.

"I think you've hit it," I said, shaking my head. "'Mysterious ways' indeed."

I removed the heating pad and castor oil pack. It must have been my imagination, but I thought those two lumps looked *smaller.*

"I feel better, Mom," David said. "My stomach isn't so tight now." His speech was a little slurred. The tranquilizer was still working on him—he was beginning to doze off.

He said that he wanted us to stay in the room with him until he was asleep. Marianne and I sat on each side of the bed. David was lying on his back. It was the only position that allowed him to sleep comfortably. Marianne was holding his hand and gently stroking his head. I held his other hand.

My, but he looks so much older than his twenty-five years.

There was no sound in David's room except our breathing. Marianne let out a little sigh. She reached for my other hand and smiled. David was drifting back into sleep. Silence. Marianne and I gazed at each other over his sleeping body. There was incredible pain in her eyes. There was also, as a strange companion to the pain, an expression of unshakable peace. I took it into myself and for a moment felt the indescribable pain of a mother losing her son. I felt Marianne and saw through her eyes. I've often wondered if it were transmitted to me because Marianne, I, and David were holding hands. It doesn't matter what form revelation takes—the importance is in the message.

It was one of those rare occasions when I would cry in front of Marianne and David, and it was a freeing feeling. No one voiced to stop me nor told me it was going to be all right. I cried for the man lying in this bed, for his mother, and for myself for being a part of it. A witness, not an outsider. I cried because along with the enormous pain and loss Marianne was feeling, I glimpsed the essence of her faith. When the soul is aroused, the body—too small and finite to express the full effect of the soul—sheds tears. In a moment I experienced what enabled her to go on. It was nothing more nor less than what I had believed and rested upon myself: a fortress, a refuge, built upon a promise, "I am with you always, even unto the end." Marianne not only believed His words true, she relied upon them to enable her to rise each morning and face the day and David's general decline in health.

I cried because I had never faced such a thing in all my life. It was so momentous and startling and new. And oh, I was beginning to love David and this family. I felt so much a part of this family much too soon. Now the flowers he was growing! It was like having the world in your hand for just a moment and then having to let it go.

But I don't have to let it go yet. Not yet, please.

There was peace in this room. Marianne was smiling, serene. When she could smile in the face of all this, I knew I could be strong for her and David. Yet I was still awed. Who could be other than solemn under these circumstances? Only someone attuned to the unchangeable essence of Spirit.

Kahlil Gibran in his book *Jesus the Son of Man* wrote: *"Have you ever heard a thrush sing while its nest burns in the wind? Have you ever seen a woman whose sorrow is too much for tears, or a wounded heart that would rise beyond its own pain?"*

Marianne did rise above and beyond the pain and came over to be a comfort to *me.* We were in this together, all of us.

We stayed with David for a long time in that silence. Marianne and I watched and waited.

16

◆

I had been visiting David for about two weeks when I finally announced the real nature of his illness to my parents. My folks and I were having dinner shortly before Christmas when I told them that I was caring for a person not with cancer, but with AIDS. We had never discussed AIDS, except in relation to Ryan White. They were sympathetic to Ryan's plight and agreed that Kokomo was overreacting, but my own involvement with someone with AIDS produced a different reaction.

"David doesn't have cancer," I told them. "He has AIDS. Arthur Martin assigned me to him because we live in the same town and he needs someone close by."

My father was alarmed.

"AIDS?" he asked, incredulous. "He's got AIDS? How do you know you can't catch it from him? They don't know everything about this disease—"

This time I interrupted. "Dad, I've read a lot about AIDS. It's transmitted through sexual activity and blood to blood contact. I wear gloves if David gets sick and vomits. I take precautions." An awkward silence followed as we ate.

Then Dad asked, "How do you know you won't come down with this disease ten years from now from being around him?"

"How do I know I won't get hit by a bus tomorrow?" I replied.

I started again, trying to be calm. "Dad, you've seen the news reports about Ryan White. That kind of thing is happening all over the country. These people need help. They're being treated like lepers."

"Somebody's got to help them. I said I would help David. We were in school together, Dad. I knew him before he got AIDS."

"How did he contract it?" Dad asked.

"It could have been a blood transfusion." David had had a transfusion some years before, after an auto accident. But I knew that David believed he had contracted it sexually.

"At this point, does it matter?" I asked. "He's very sick and needs help. That's all I'm concerned about."

We continued to eat dinner in silence. Finally, Mom said she was glad I was involved and glad of what I was doing.

"I'm proud of you for wanting to help. Like I said before, it takes a special breed of people to take care of those who are very sick and dying. We're just worried, honey," she said. "They really don't know all there is to know about AIDS yet. Your dad is just expressing a natural fear any parent would have in this situation. We just want you to be careful."

I could understand her point of view. If I were a parent, I would be worried about my kid—even having the facts about AIDS in front of me.

"I'm sorry if I was defensive," I said. "It's just that I've watched the horrible treatment of those with AIDS on the news, like Ryan. It gets my hackles up when people think AIDS is caught like a cold. It's not. Science has proven that much. AIDS is practically impossible to contract under casual conditions."

"But this isn't casual," Dad said. "Taking care of him when he's sick is not casual contact."

"No, I guess it's not," I said. "But this is important to me, and I can't really say why. It's something I have to do."

We didn't explore the "I can't really say why" part of the conversation. I didn't tell my parents that I had wrestled not only with the issues of death and dying, but also the dilemma of my own sexuality for most of my life. I'd known I was gay since my early teens. I felt I couldn't talk to my parents about my sexual orientation because I didn't understand it. Homosexuality was a subject I'd never heard of nor read about in my early teens. I suppressed it at the time because I was convinced something was very wrong with me. I was silent not only with my parents, but my closest friends didn't know of my secret.

Around the age of fourteen, I convinced myself that I was going through a phase that would eventually pass. When I came to the realization that it was not a phase, not going away, that's when I began a search for deeper understanding and meaning in life. When I first became aware of my homosexuality, the "traveling minister's" words haunted me. I thought I was bad and sinful. I knew I was different, but didn't know why. I carried it like a heavy weight throughout my teen-age years and early adulthood. Even with the evidence of the early comforting experiences in meditation and the "all is well" message that came to me, I still felt ill at ease in dealing with this alien part of my psyche.

It wasn't until I joined the navy that I met other gay people who had also struggled with their own homosexuality. My eventual acceptance of being gay came only after a long period of inner struggle and turmoil, after a lot of reading, searching, and talking with gay people from all walks of life. I eventually surrendered to the fact that I could not change this part of myself any more than I could change the color of my eyes.

In retrospect, I could see that I went through the five stages terminally ill patients go through in the eventual acceptance of their death. Initially, I denied that homosexuality would be an integral part of the rest of my life: it was a phase; it was going to go away. It was my dark secret, and I was alone with it. The complement—or should I say curse?—to the first stage of denial is isolation. In my aloneness, I turned to keeping a journal. I could express in writing, in private, the things I could never speak of openly. My love for writing was indeed borne of great inner conflict.

Then came the anger. This "phase" wasn't passing. I was angry at God, at nature, at life. Why was I different? Why couldn't I be like other people? Why me? What was the reason for my being gay? These unanswerable questions created a quick, flaring temper in my teen-age years. The frustration that I felt in being so alone with my homosexuality made me angrier still. The anger was an unresolved issue even throughout my time with David. An outlet for that anger was against the insensitive treatment of people with AIDS. The injustices touched off my inner anger and flourished. The subject was closer to home with me than anyone knew.

I also went through the third stage of "bargaining" in my teen years. I thought if I prayed long enough, hard enough, and was good enough, God would bless me with a "normal" heterosexual life.

The depression set in when my prayers were not answered. I feel that it drove me to seek to understand life beyond the three dimensions. Beyond my fears of death, I believe my inability to deal with my homosexuality led me to search and eventually find the Cayce material as well as other books.

Acceptance of my sexuality came only after I *did* discover the metaphysical sciences. The concept of reincarnation was of great help to me in understanding my sexual nature. Cayce had often said that "life is a continuous experience" and that we come to the earth as a school to "experience all things." I saw that perhaps my homosexuality was a part of my soul's journey through time and space. Hugh Lynn had said that who we are today is a sum total of all of our lives, all of our experiences—now. My sum total was expressing itself perhaps near androgeny—the harmony between the male and female aspects of the soul. I am expressing more of the feminine aspects of my soul, as a man. I was and am completely happy being a man in this lifetime; my mind, however, expresses the intuitive, or the feminine, through my male self. A unique expression, to be sure, but one that caused me a great deal of confusion for many years.

Years after my time in the navy, I sought a deeper understanding of my homosexuality and began the process of psychotherapy with a Jungian analyst. He taught me that all creativity comes from the receptive or feminine side of the mind and soul. My being drawn to the arts, writing, and service-oriented professions was an aspect of the feminine side of my soul's manifestation. I knew that some of the great artists of all time were gay: Michelangelo, da Vinci, Walt Whitman, Tennessee Williams. I came to understand that my being gay was a natural consequence of expressing these feminine aspects of the soul as a man. It was the exception rather than the rule; there are scores of gifted artists and thinkers who are heterosexual.

These concepts made sense and were liberating to me. Homosexuality remains a mystery to science and medicine. Great debates had been held throughout the centuries as to its origin. No solid or lasting understanding became clear to me until I considered homosexuality from the spiritual perspective of the ongoing development of the soul. I was freed when I truly felt my nature to be an expression of my soul's evolution and not a genetic malfunction nor a result of a dysfunctional family.

I concluded that my homosexuality was an aspect of my soul's manifestation in the earth—not the *only* facet, but *one.* Many friends have told me that they came to a greater understanding about homosexuality through meeting and coming to know me. I believe that is one of the reasons I entered this life gay: to shed a new light upon the metaphysical aspects of homosexuality.

I also believe that my being gay drew me to eventually be with David and want to help people with AIDS. In many ways my ministry to him helped me to come to terms with my own sexuality as well, not just the issues of death and dying. Perhaps one of the reasons I entered this lifetime as a homosexual was to help people like David who was gay and attempt to shed light in the wake of great ignorance. If I had been born a heterosexual, I've wondered if I would have become involved with people with AIDS. It's difficult to gauge what my life would have been like had I been heterosexual. I've wondered if I would have had the sensitivity to care for gay men with AIDS and want to take an active role in helping them at a very intimate level and time of their lives. I doubt it.

In the wake of the AIDS epidemic, it was natural for me to want to help my own: It could have easily been I who was a patient instead of a support person.

These deeper reasons for my involvement with David had never surfaced in family discussions. But I believe intuitively that my mother and father knew. It did not, in the end, matter. My parents came to care for David and his family a great deal and were sympathetic and supportive. After I had been helping him and his family for a month, David began to frequently telephone and talk with Mom. They had gardening in common; David talked about all his exotic plants. He became endeared to Mom. He had the personality of those individuals who've never met a stranger. People liked him immediately. Mom was no exception.

When my folks learned of what David, as well as Marianne, had gone through in the past year, there was a shift in their attitude. They were empathetic and began to worry less about me contracting AIDS and became more concerned for David. It was a period of great relief for me.

Mom began to save newspaper articles about the latest medical updates on AIDS. After a while, it became easy for Mom, Dad, and me to talk about the epidemic and the plight of people with AIDS.

One day when I came home from work, Mom handed me the daily newspaper of Morgan.

"You're not going to be happy about this," she said.

The newspaper editor, who regularly labeled homosexuals "perverts" in the headlines of the daily Morgan newspaper, had written an editorial about gay people and AIDS. It was scathing and hurtful. My effort not to be angered by media ignorance was forgotten when the editor added people with AIDS to his list of "perverts."

The editor was acquainted with Marianne and David and was well aware that David had AIDS. His callousness made me furious. When I went to David's that evening, a copy of the newspaper was on the dining room table. David was resting, and Marianne was in tears looking at the paper.

"Why, Rob? Why would he write this? He knows me. He knows David. This just kills me." She left the table crying and went into her room. Lillian was in the living room. I sat down by her.

"People are so cruel," Lillian said. "Poor David. It's bad enough he is suffering so. But the article in the paper! Horrible. Marianne has enough to deal with without this."

Lillian told me about Tricia, the woman who demanded that the board of directors of a local health spa drain the swimming pool after David had swum in it. Marianne had been friends with Tricia, had taught her daughter to swim. After Tricia forced the pool to be drained, she stopped speaking to Marianne.

Marianne at one time had many friends in the local community. Over the years she had taught most of the children in Morgan to swim. Many of those friends didn't call any more. She still taught their kids at the health center, but the parents regarded her cooly. In the AIDS epidemic, the parents of children with AIDS also become outcasts.

"I'm going to write the editor," I said finally. "I'm sick of all of this. I doubt the paper will print it, but I'm going to write him and let him know just what kind of effect he's having."

I was surprised to come home from work some weeks after mailing my response to the editor to find it printed in the paper. To the paper's credit, it was printed with minimal editing:

> I work in a support group for AIDS patients. Considering your view on AIDS, you might consider handling this letter with rubber gloves. From your article of March 17, you seem to be the type that would move your own wife onto the street if she contracted Acquired Immune Deficiency Syndrome. If she contracted it through a blood transfusion, would she be a "pervert"?
>
> Do you classify Ryan White a pervert because he contracted AIDS? . . . I have close friends in this county and in Indianapolis who are AIDS patients . . . To those who know your writing, they cannot understand your hatred. Hatred not for the disease, but to them personally.
>
> One mother of an AIDS patient read one of your ar-

ticles and burst into tears, feeling more helpless than ever, feeling more persecuted than ever. She never deserved your condemnation or your hatred. AIDS is a disease: It doesn't discriminate between blacks or whites, male or female, heterosexual or homosexual. It's a virus. A *virus.*

The way you write about this disease makes people angry. And leads them to shut themselves off from any other information on AIDS. They will remain in the dark and fearful. They will remain ignorant. Your views on AIDS inspires people to throw rocks and bottles at the homes of AIDS patients.

People with AIDS are still people. They are sick people like cancer patients who still need love and care and hope. If you'll not think of the patients, think of the mothers, the relatives, the friends of AIDS victims. They do not deserve your wrath. They do not deserve to be condemned. Especially the mothers. The hardest thing in the world for parents to do is witness the slow death of their child. And you are condemning them when you have no right to condemn.

These people, regardless of their sexual orientation, are people with a disease. And I do not understand why you kick them when they are already down. Aren't they suffering enough without your "help"?

Beneath my letter, the editor wrote: "For the victim, pity; for the disease, hate." There were no further editorial comments in the Letters to the Editor section.

An amazing thing happened as a result of my letter. The editor stopped referring to homosexuals or people with AIDS as "perverts" in headlines or editorials.

I had warned my parents I was writing the letter. They were supportive, but fearful of a backlash from the local community. Surprisingly, there was no negative response.

In fact, a Catholic priest called our home and talked to my mother, saying my letter was "long overdue." He said he had been despondent by the editor's scathing editorials for a long time.

"You should be very proud of your son for writing that letter," the priest told my mother.

Mom was very excited about the priest's telephone call. I was excited to see her excitement! It wasn't long after that that my parents began to talk to their friends and our relatives about David, Ryan White, and AIDS. They were supportive and open and helped dispel some of the fear and ignorance. I spent a lot of time talking with my folks about what I had learned about AIDS.

Years later, my mother said words to me I'll never forget:

"The miracle of having kids is that eventually they teach the parents. You have."

17

◆

*M*arianne put her arms around me and gave me a big hug when I went over after my letter was published.

"Thank you for writing the letter," she said. "People have called and told me how sorry they were and offered support." Marianne was radiant. I was happy and relieved that I was able to channel my anger into a constructive outlet.

"David's lying down. He's got a surprise for you." Her eyes twinkled. "He actually has two surprises."

David was sitting up in bed when I came into his room.

"Look at this, Rob," David said and held up a charcoal sketching of a landscape. It was beautiful. "I had a good day today," he said. "I haven't felt this good in a long time."

"I love it, David," I said. "God, I wish that I could sketch like that." I marveled at his ability to stay creative. In the

short time I had known David, I had learned a valuable lesson about strength, about courage, and about facing life
even against unbeatable odds. His condition didn't stop
him from drawing or playing music or gardening. He didn't
give up on *life*. Could I ever muster such courage? I wondered if I would have the strength to even get out of bed
were I in his shoes.

"That's a very nice surprise," I said.

"No, that's not the surprise," David said. "Look."

David lifted up his T-shirt and revealed his abdomen. "No
lumps," he said. "Your castor oil is amazing."

I was incredulous. The two walnut-sized lumps I had
seen when I placed the castor oil pack on his stomach were
indeed gone. David was smiling. I'd never seen him look
happier. "I've used the pack every day for the last week. The
pressure is down a lot, too," he said.

"He's kept his food down for two days." I turned around
and Marianne was standing in the doorway. "I don't know
what's in those packs," she said. "Whatever it is, David is
feeling a whole lot better. Thank God."

I was speechless! I looked closely at David's stomach. The
swelling from his liver was down as well. I had read a lot of
amazing accounts of the success of castor oil packs. This
was the first time I'd ever seen them work.

"I felt good enough today that I did some composing at
the piano," David said and handed me a cassette tape. "I
want you to hear it." Such a change in David! He was still
very ill, but his eyes looked clearer and his face had more
color than usual.

I put the tape in the cassette player beside his bed and sat
down in a lotus position against the wall. David lay back
and closed his eyes.

"Close your eyes," David said. "I want you to really take
this in."

The music began with David playing one note over and

over. Then began a lilting melody, reminiscent of the Pachabel Canon. Soon, it sounded as if David were playing every key on the piano; the sound of a musical waterfall. There were three distinct pieces on the tape, but without a pause; they blended well. Chills crept up my back and neck as I listened to David's composition. It was fluid and haunting. He played straight through the thirty-minute cassette without hitting an off-key and without a break.

I'm in the presence of something divine.

This thought was a surety, a knowing. The same knowing was characteristic of what I had experienced several times in meditation, as well as on the hill of Golgotha in Jerusalem. I kept my eyes closed and sailed on the rhythms of David's music. It was simply magic. Another of the almost-mystical realizations stole over me, inspired by David's music:

God works and moves through us.

The music built to a climax. In my mind's eye, I could clearly see David seated at the piano, eyes closed, playing. Above him I could see a source of bright light—a shining, creative Force—luminescent and brilliant—moving through him, using him as a channel. The form was a glowing liquid, its movement above and around David was a dance. It poured through the top of his head, filling him. As this energy form moved through him, it rippled out from his fingertips. At first I thought this form was moving to the rhythm of the musical notes. Then I realized it was creating the musical notes. At the points of his fingertips on the piano keys, I could see the result of the light movement: the music.

God moves through us. That's what I'm seeing.

In David's room, in this space and time, it was not strange to have such a vision. It was not a peculiar happening among the blooming spring flowers in the dead of winter. It was not bizarre at all among the silent sentinels of David's picture-perfect sketches and paintings surrounding me, created by a person who could barely walk. To the outside world of appearances, yes, it was strange—even miraculous—to hear such music when the musician's body was a mere shadow. But here, in this moment with David, the miracles were simply a part of life and living—and yes, even of death and dying.

I was seeing that although David was dying, some other part of him was vitally alive. It made no difference that his body was wasting away; his spirit was becoming more vibrant, more tangible. The body was racked with pain, slowly shutting itself down, the soul made up for the pain by expressing itself passionately, almost urgently.

The crescendo of music slowly wound down to a quieter interlude. The river of music became a stream, then a trickle, then a drop. The piece ended as it had begun: with one note.

"My gift to you," David said, opening his eyes.

I didn't trust my voice. "I don't know what to say."

David did not move, only smiled. His eyes were almost hypnotic. The faraway look was more prominent now.

He did not take his gaze off me. What I saw in his eyes I can only express as David in gradual transition from this world. I also saw the brilliance of that part of him that played the music—totally untouched by his dying body. He was thoughtful, his voice almost a whisper when he spoke.

"I read your letter to the paper, Rob. Thanks. That helped my mom a lot."

I nodded my head, not speaking; feeling at peace in David's room with the blooming flowers, the paintings, the vibrations of his music still surrounding me. I felt strange, not uncomfortably so, with the nearness of the forces of life and death.

"I'm beginning to feel myself letting go," David said. "But I'm not ready just yet."

I realized I had written of death in my letter to the editor. There was a moment of pain when I realized I had written, "The hardest thing in the world for parents to do is witness the slow death of their child." Then I became aware that David was not anxious about it and didn't appear afraid.

"It's O.K. now," he said, still gazing at me with his hypnotic eyes. "I was afraid it was going to hurt all the way to the end. It's not, really. Sometimes I get the feeling as if I'm going down a long hill from real high up."

"Are you scared?" I asked.

"No. Well, sometimes. I have good days and bad days when I think about it. Right now, no, I'm not."

I asked David if he minded if I recorded our conversation. It suddenly seemed very important that I preserve our discussion. At the time, I didn't know why. He agreed, and he told me where his blank cassette tapes were kept. I took his music tape out of the player and put in the blank cassette. David watched me intently as I went about to record our conversation.

"Do you know what I call that musical piece?" he asked. "'Sunrise Trilogy.' It came out of me in three segments, all strung together. I made it up as I played."

"David, how do you feel when you play like that? I had an unusual experience while I was listening to it."

"I feel as if God is playing through me," he said. "I ask Him to. I think He does."

"I think He does, too," I said. It was eerie that David was speaking of my vision. What I had seen of the light-energy-force was real. I told him what I had seen while I was listening to his music.

"I've always tried to allow that to happen," David said. "I've always believed that God comes through me when I paint or play music. But I've never felt it so powerful before.

"That's how I know I'm dying," he added.

I looked at him a long time before I spoke. "David, you

know, I read something once that said 'The body is a hindrance to the soul at times.' "

"I'll be glad to get rid of it, actually." Suddenly, we both started laughing. "I've just about worn this one out," he added in his comical way.

"I hate to talk in clichés, Dave," I said, "but somebody said, 'There are greater worlds than these.' I know there are. This is but a shadow of the real life in the spiritual realms."

"Do you really think so? I'm beginning to believe that. I have dreams sometimes. I've been dreaming of people who have died. Friends, relatives. The dreams seem more real than right now. Is that weird?"

Cayce had said in a reading that the dream state is a shadow of the place we go at death. He also said that when we dream of departed loved ones, it is more than a dream. In some way, we are in contact with them.

"No, it's not weird at all," I told him. "I think it's a sort of preparation for you. In the same way that we've got doctors and nurses to help us be born here on the earth, I think there are the souls of people we've known that help us over to the 'other side.' "

"Do you think it will hurt?" he asked. "When I go, I mean. Do you think that final plunge is painful?"

"Remember what Janie said at the support group? I think she's right. This is the hard part, living right up to the time of the transition."

"That's what it is, isn't it?" David asked. "A transition?"

"Yes," I said. "That's all it is. A change of place."

"I used to worry a lot about hell and being damned," David remembered, as he sat up with some difficulty.

"So did I," I replied, and told him about the minister I had met in my preteen years. "I used to lie awake at night and worry about my parents being 'saved.' Then I used to worry about me being 'saved.' It screwed me up for a good many years."

"Me, too," David answered. "I think the idea of eternal damnation is like God cutting off His arm. We're part of God. He can't destroy or separate Himself, can He?"

"No, I don't think so. There's one of the Psalms I love. 'Though I take on the wings of morning and fly to the utmost parts of the universe, Thou art there. Though I may make my bed in hell, behold, Thou art there.' (Psalm 139) I believe that God is everywhere. I read once that each of us— each soul—is a corpuscle in the body of God. We're part of God. We can't be damned."

"I believe that, too," David said. "Why do you think people see God in such a negative way? All this eternal damnation stuff."

I was thoughtful. "I think back in the biblical days the teachers threatened people so they would act right. Maybe it was the only way they would listen."

"Maybe," David responded. "I don't think I'm going to hell. I've done plenty I'm sorry for, but I've also done a lot I'm happy about."

I thought about David's creativity. "I think all the things you do so beautifully, the plants, the music, the art—all those things are reassurances that—in a spiritual sense— you're doing just fine."

"I get that feeling. It's just scary. I can't be sure about anything. There's no proof of heaven or hell or whatever. But I feel that God is preparing me. It's weird that the plants bloom the way they do. And my music! I've always played— but it's like now it's effortless. When I feel that—I really feel that God loves me."

David began to doze. I sat with him until he went into a deep sleep.

I got up and once again looked at the flowers, the paintings, and the sketches, still amazed.

"He does love you, David. More than you know."

18

◆

*T*he support group meetings in Indianapolis became a highlight of David's week. He was growing close to several people in the group and loved to socialize. He was very disappointed when he didn't feel well enough to attend every meeting, but we usually went to the group every other Monday evening. I would drive up to the door of Dan's office, while Arthur or another member of the group would help David from the car into the meeting room. Although he moved very slowly and painfully, he was determined to attend group as long as he didn't feel nauseous and his temperature didn't rise above 102 degrees.

Arthur began exploring creative visualization in the support group. One Monday evening, we all watched a videotape of one of Louise Hay's workshops. Her work in California was becoming increasingly popular throughout

the country. She believed that through creative mental visualization or attitude "reprogramming"—changing a
negative self-image to a positive and loving outlook—
people could heal themselves. It was a philosophy that echoed Edgar Cayce's view that mind is the builder and that
which we dwell upon, we become.

Louise Hay's guided meditations were powerful and
emotional. While participants were in a relaxed, lightly hypnotic state, Louise gently suggested affirmations on self-
love and peace, and, most important, she helped people let
go of their guilt and shame. She taught self-empowerment,
that we must learn to accept and forgive ourselves for our
shortcomings.

The sessions had a profound effect upon David. They
helped him feel stronger physically, and he was able to let
go of a great deal of negativity and guilt. David was prone to
bouts of severe depression. He told me he often felt responsible for putting his family "through hell." The hell David
referred to was his growing dependency on his family's care
as he got worse. He found comfort and a sense of healing in
Louise Hay's words.

David's depression was normal. Dan had said that anytime a person is sick physically, there sometimes is a mental
clouding in which he or she feels unproductive and sad. I
thought David did very, very well under the circumstances.

Seeing him in a bright state of mind or seeing him free of
pain and happy was a grand occasion. I noticed that those
occasions became more frequent after the guided meditations with the support group. David and I decided to work
with creative visualization and guided meditations at home.
The sessions became a regular routine. I would play music
very low—many times we used David's own music for the
sessions. While he was lying in bed, I would verbally help
him to relax every part of his body, beginning with his toes
and moving to the top of his head. After he was in a com-

pletely relaxed state, I would start with Louise Hay's suggestions that David was surrounded in white light and that it was moving through him, healing and relaxing every part of his body. Over and over, I would tell him that every organ in his body was functioning perfectly and he was at complete peace.

I suggested using the white light for reasons beyond relaxation. I hoped that he could visualize the light that people had so often seen in near-death experiences. I hoped that at the point of his transition the coming light would be familiar to him, and it would be easy for him to let go. I also thought that perhaps the light might bring a physical healing. My mind was open that anything was possible.

Since David had so much trouble sleeping at night, I usually wouldn't bring him out of the sleep state at the end of the sessions, but would suggest that he drift into a natural, restful sleep.

After one of the visualization sessions, I went into the living room to talk with Lillian, Marianne, and her sister-in-law Gayle, who was visiting from Florida. David and Gayle were very close. Marianne often said that David was the male counterpart of Gayle and vice versa. When I met her, I saw many similarities. She had a sharp wit, a vivacious personality, and she was quick to laugh. I was drawn to her immediately.

David had been looking forward to her visit for weeks. They talked and laughed and shared stories. AIDS was not a stumbling block for Gayle. She lived in Florida where the AIDS-awareness and education campaigns were very visible.

Gayle was another of those people who never met a stranger. She had the quality, like David, that made you feel as if you'd known her for years.

"How is he doing?" Gayle asked.

I told her about the guided meditations and Louise Hay.

"Those sessions are helping David to sleep," I answered. "I hope it's doing more good than that, but at least he can sleep now."

"Thank God," Lillian said.

"That's the worst part of this whole thing," Marianne added. "He has those high fevers that just sap the energy out of him. But he can't sleep unless he's heavily sedated. He doesn't need the pills so often when Rob leads him through these relaxation sessions."

I told her I would make a recording of one of the sessions so that she could play it when I wasn't there.

"I believe in all that," Gayle remarked. "I've been looking into a lot of different alternative therapies."

"For David?" I asked.

"For me," Gayle replied. At those words, Marianne put her hand on Gayle's shoulder. I was puzzled.

"The doctors have given Gayle six months to live," Lillian stated.

I was shocked. I looked at Gayle—radiant, happy. Her piercing blue eyes looked at me with a mix of confusion. But her expression held no fear and she spoke matter of factly before I could inquire.

"It started out as a pain in the rib," Gayle said, indicating her lower right side. "Then my hip started bothering me. After a thorough exam and a bone marrow sample was taken, the doctors said I've got cancer."

I shook my head in disbelief. "Gayle, I don't know what to say. I'm so sorry."

"Hey, don't worry about it," Gayle said. "I think the doctors are crazy. Oh, I can believe about the cancer, but this six months' stuff is crap." She reached for a cigarette. "Here's the real clincher: They told me it has spread everywhere but my lungs." I lit my own cigarette as well as Gayle's. "I just can't believe it," she added.

I asked her about getting a second or a third opinion.

"I just got back from Sloan-Kettering," Gayle said. "I went to the head honchos. They're the ones who gave me the death sentence."

"Don't say that!" Marianne replied sharply. She wasn't in the mood for dark humor.

"Oh, me and my big mouth! I'm sorry, Marianne. You know me, though, I don't pull punches." Gayle looked over at me. "I told David if I could trade places with him, I would. I'm getting around a hell of a lot better than he is. Poor kid."

It wasn't a matter of Gayle being in a state of denial over her diagnosis—she simply felt too good for such a prognosis to be true. She still played tennis three times a week and ran a plumbing business that had turned into a small empire. She also did volunteer work on the side.

"The pain is slowly getting worse," Gayle said, "but it hasn't stopped me."

I felt very open with Gayle and recommended some books by Elisabeth Kübler-Ross. I also told her more about Louise Hay's work.

"I'm not afraid of death," Gayle said. "It's the process of dying that scares me." Marianne put her arms around Gayle.

"We've gone through too much together for me to lose you now," Marianne said. Gayle's husband, Marianne's brother, had died of a heart attack less than two years before. Prior to that, Lillian's husband, Marianne's father, had died after a long battle with cancer. Marianne and Lillian had cared for him in their home until he died.

Lillian sighed and looked out the window. "Yes, God knows we have gone through a lot."

Gayle laughed despite the darkness of the moment and, with Marianne still holding her, said: "Ever get the feeling we've been cursed?"

Marianne turned her attention to me. "What is it you say, Rob? Are we cleaning up our karma, or what?"

"I think you all have graduated," I said. "After this life, you all get a one-way ticket to heaven!"

"I'll drink to that," Gayle exclaimed.

"Me, too," Marianne replied.

"Me, three," Lillian added.

We all got up from the living room and made our way to the kitchen to fix drinks.

I took in the scene like a photographer. These three women had been called to endure what the outside world would call immense tragedy. As always, I wondered what was going on in the spiritual sense. Appearances often defied what was being developed at the spiritual level. I thought of a passage from Richard Bach's book, *Illusions*:

> "The mark of your ignorance is the depth of your belief in injustice and tragedy.
>
> "What the caterpillar calls the end of the world, the master calls a butterfly."

We raised our glasses to one another.

"Here's to good friends and family," I said, toasting.

"And to life," Gayle said. "May it never end."

19

◆

O ne evening at the close of the guided meditation, David spoke with a sense of urgency. He usually fell deeply asleep during the session. As I got up to join Marianne in the living room, David startled me by speaking from a semi-conscious state.

"I want to meet your parents. Especially your dad."

I turned, expecting David to be awake. David was asleep. It caught me quite off guard.

"Please, Rob. Soon." I looked closely at David's face. His eyes were moving back and forth beneath his closed lids. He was in the "dream" state! Where did his words come from? He uttered them in the monotone voice of the sleeping. It was familiar; I'd heard my brothers talk in their sleep when we were kids.

David had said on more than one occasion that he had

admired my father's work when we were in high school. Dad not only taught machine shop, but also taught mechanical drawing, auto mechanics, and woodworking. He also dabbled in oil and watercolor painting, giving away many of his paintings, but several portraits were still in our home. It was interesting that David shared the talents of my mother's ability to garden and my father's ability to paint.

As David lay sleeping, I thought of the many things he had in common with my parents. In his back yard, he had built an elevated garden using railroad ties. The ties were arranged in a triangular shape about five feet high. He filled it with earth and planted flowers in the spring of each year. Like David, Dad had also built elevated gardens for Mom in front of our home. In the corner of David's yard, he had created a rock garden around his rose bushes. The roses flourished there. I had seen pictures of his outdoor gardens, but had yet to see them in bloom.

David wanted to meet my parents. True, they had common interests, but I didn't understand the urgency. His words, spoken from a subconscious state, haunted me: *Please, Rob. Soon.* They told me that time was short. They left the impression on me of ending and completion. A feeling very much as one feels when autumn is in the air at the close of summer.

How close was David to his transition? Physically, the evidence of his being near death was clear; he was moving slower with each passing day, and he was progressively losing more weight. There had been no new infections or ailments, however. But my feeling went beyond his physical deterioration. I could feel that David was needing to wrap things up in this world, be about what Elisabeth Kübler-Ross called "unfinished business." Part of that business included meeting my family.

When I asked David the following day if he remembered telling me he wanted to meet my folks, he was surprised.

"I don't remember saying that," he replied, "but I do want to meet them. That is, if they want to meet me." From his deep, unconscious state of mind, David had been able to convey something he couldn't bring himself to say consciously. Perhaps he was afraid that I would deny his request to meet my folks. He had grown close to Mom, but had never really talked to Dad.

I told David about my folks' initial reaction to the news that I was spending time with people with AIDS. But time had changed them, and I knew my parents would want to meet David. It was March 1986—only a few months since I had told them David had AIDS. But we all had grown in that short time. Mom and Dad and I talked of David, as well as Marianne and Lillian, as members of our family. Mom even got in the habit of asking about "Grandma" instead of "Lillian."

I knew David would have to meet my family soon. He was getting worse by the day. The continued castor oil packs were helping him to keep down the small amount of food he consumed. The packs also helped alleviate the abdominal pressure. The strange lumps I had seen on his abdomen never appeared again. But the chronic active hepatitis made the cells of the liver proliferate to cover the damaged cells. The enlargement of the liver was the result. His coughing became worse, and he began to cough up blood.

It had been less than two years since David traveled to Florida and California. He had been a model, a body-builder, living a very independent life. The hardest part for him was his reliance on others for help with the simplest tasks. He had to be assisted to and from the table for meals. He could no longer drive a car. Dependency was a major issue in the support group as well. "Attaboy" John was also getting weaker and was frustrated that it took so much time for him to merely walk up the stairs to his apartment. I found the loss of all independence the most brutal aspect of AIDS. Eventually most all AIDS patients become bedridden.

On some days, David needed assistance in walking around the house. His ankles and feet were badly swollen, causing a great deal of pain. The headaches were worse, requiring more narcotics. David would periodically have his blood work done at the Indiana University Medical Center in Indianapolis. The most recent tests showed the presence of an "unknown" virus that was wreaking havoc in his bloodstream. The presence of the HIV was killing his immune system, but this other volatile bug that modern science had never seen was attacking his red blood cells. Raging fevers—sometimes as high as 104 degrees—were the result.

Physicians had told Marianne that David would eventually need blood transfusions because his body wouldn't produce the needed blood cells. The tuberculosis of the bone marrow was hindering the natural process of blood creation. David continued to lose weight when it seemed there wasn't anything more of him to lose. Remarkably, however, he had not contracted the *Pneumocystis carinii pneumonia* nor the Kaposi's sarcoma—the two prevalent opportunistic infections that attack most people with AIDS. That was little comfort in the wake of everything else David was suffering.

If people who were ignorant and fearful about AIDS met David, their views would change. If people could see a twenty-five-year-old become an old man overnight, perhaps they would understand how difficult, how horrific AIDS is.

Yet, AIDS did indeed present an opportunity to learn how precious and fragile life is. David had become a teacher for me. More than anything, I was inspired by his stamina. He kept on going by sheer will alone. He continued living for the simple and the ordinary. He had one wish, one desire that enabled him to carry on: He wanted to see the spring one more time. Through the winter months, he had looked forward to the coming of spring as a child awaits Christmas. He had created spring in his very own house with his plants and flowers, but it was not enough.

"I'm hanging on for spring," he said to me once. "I've got to see my flowers and roses bloom outside." In the weekly visualization sessions, I would suggest that David see himself outside amid the flowers and trees in bloom. Roses were his favorite flower, so I would tell him to picture the roses in full bloom. Often when we began the visualization sessions, David was exhausted or in pain. By the time I had relaxed him and asked him to see the flowers, he was noticeably more at ease. There was relief on his face. Respite from physical pain was a precious gift in David's last months. I'm glad there were moments when he was comfortable and free from pain.

Every day Marianne, Lillian, and I were reminded that AIDS was slowly but surely taking David, a piece at a time. A person in the latter stages of AIDS, as David was, had no idea what the day would bring. He lived in a state of dread, never knowing when the AIDS symptoms would overcome him.

In a twenty-four-hour period, David would be able to keep his food down, be in minimal pain, exude high energy, laugh and joke with us, and sleep through the night. In the next twenty-four hours, his temperature would rise, in a matter of hours, to 103 degrees. He would be overcome with violent diarrhea lasting most of the day, leaving him dehydrated and exhausted. He would suffer excruciating headaches and remain bedridden, but sleepless, for the entire night. The pain in his joints and bones disabled him so that he couldn't walk. When he finally did sleep, the night sweats would soak the sheets and blankets of his bed and they'd have to be changed in the middle of the night. These attacks became more frequent as the days wore on.

David hated hospitals. He would fight Marianne tooth and nail when he had to go. Marianne would take David to the hospital when his fevers wouldn't go down. Usually it required several days of intravenous antibiotics. Sometimes during his weekly checkups at the I.U. Medical Center, the attending physician would admit David for several days of observation.

When people with AIDS talk about "good and bad days," I was witnessing just how good and how bad they can be.

I waited for one of David's good days to take him to my parents' house. Mom and Dad welcomed the opportunity to meet him. When I told my folks that David wanted to visit, they didn't hesitate.

"Bring him out," Dad said.

"We'd love to have him," Mom added.

I tried to brace my parents for meeting David; I knew his physical condition would be shocking. His appearance sometimes affected me deeply, even though I had gone beyond knowing David simply as a person with AIDS; I had gotten to know him as a friend and saw the inner part of him.

Winter was still in full force when Marianne and I bundled up David to visit my house. We gathered an arsenal of his medicines to take along, in case he was nauseous or in more pain than usual.

"Oh, wait," David said. "I almost forgot. I want to take your Mom a start from my spider plant." He snapped one of the "babies" off the hanging planter and wrapped it in a paper towel.

As David and I said our good-bys to his mother and grandmother, I remembered the first night I had taken him to the support group. It seemed like a hundred years ago. I held onto his arm and shoulders, and we made our way slowly to my car.

"I can remember running out to meet my friends as we

walked to school," David remarked. There was great sadness in his voice.

"What happened?" he asked, suddenly. I had opened the passenger side door and was helping him into the car when he stopped, holding onto me tightly. "Rob—what happened that things had to go like this?"

We stood together in the winter evening, looking into each other's eyes. I had no answer to David's question. I shook my head but didn't turn away from his questioning gaze. He suddenly hugged me fiercely, and I did the only thing I knew how to do—I hugged him back. I could see Marianne standing in the doorway, watching us. I waved her back in the house and nodded that everything was all right.

Come quickly, spring. Please—come quickly—for David.

David slowly let go of me, and I helped him into the car. He was wiping away tears as I closed the passenger door. As I got in, David was apologetic. He wasn't a physically demonstrative person, as far as hugging goes. When he did need a hug, I knew he was feeling either emotionally or physically distraught.

"I'm sorry," David apologized. "Sometimes I just wish I could understand it all. I wish I had answers."

"It's O.K.," I said. "You don't have to apologize, David. I wish I had the answers for you. I'm sorry I don't."

We drove the three-mile trip to my house mostly in silence. As we were turning into the driveway, he said, "I've looked forward to this, Rob. Thanks for bringing me."

"Do me a favor?" he asked. He looked a bit embarrassed. "Help me up the steps, but let me walk in the house myself. I want to meet your parents without being helped—I need to meet them on my own."

"Sure, Dave." I understood it was important for him to show them he was still functioning on his own. It was as if he wanted to tell the world, *AIDS has got me—but it hasn't beaten me.*

I helped him up the steps, opened the door, and let him walk in unassisted. Mom was in the kitchen, finishing up the evening's dishes. David walked ever so slowly, with the gait of an old man, to meet my mother.

I introduced them formally, even though they had met over the telephone. Mom came into the foyer as David slowly, painfully made his way to close the distance between them, his hand outstretched.

"It is a pleasure, Mrs. Grant." David was beaming. "I've waited a long time to meet you."

"I'm glad you're here, David." Mom was smiling and gracious. She offered him a seat and asked if he wanted a drink. David shook his head politely.

"I want to meet Mr. Grant."

"Oh, of course!" Mom said. "He's in the—"

Before she could finish the sentence, David was ambling through the kitchen and heading for the living room. Mom and I looked at each other in amused surprise. Typical of David, he wasn't waiting for directions or an introduction. Before I headed in David's direction, I could see the shocked and pained expression beneath the smile on my mother's face:

He's only a year older than you.

As I entered the living room, I saw a scene I never could have imagined a year before—my father standing face to face and shaking hands with a person with AIDS.

"It is an honor to meet you, Mr. Grant," David said. "I've heard so many good things about you. I've been so looking forward to meeting you."

Dad and David shook hands; it wasn't quick nor did it seem uncomfortable. Dad knew that he meant a lot to me. He had gotten used to hearing about David, and he had enjoyed learning about his gardening, painting, and music. In many ways, my father was meeting an extended member of the family. It was emotional for me to see them not merely introduce themselves and step away, but really take to each other. There was almost a tangible sense of acceptance between them. They did know one another.

Dad was very sincere when he responded, "I've heard a lot of good things about you, too. I'm really glad you came."

It was one of the last evenings of David's life when he truly felt physically and emotionally well. He didn't have any of the violent coughing spells nor did he feel in more pain than usual, and he wasn't ravaged by exhaustion. He talked easily and freely with my folks about his artwork and gardening. David was delighted that he could give my mother gardening tips and share his vast knowledge of nature with someone outside of his family.

I think the evening stands out prominently in my memory because it was a normal, pleasant visit. Days and nights with a semblance of normalcy were robbed from David because of his deteriorating physical condition. Again I was reminded just how much I took for granted in everyday life.

A highlight of that night was when David discovered the music organ in our living room.

"Oh, look!" David exclaimed. "Do you mind if I play it?" We'd had the organ for years, but none of our family ever became accomplished in music. It sat silent most of the time.

"We'd love it if you'd play us something," Mom replied.

We fetched David a pillow. Since he had very little muscle tissue left, he wasn't able to sit on hardwood chairs without one.

We sat back and listened as David played some of my parents' favorite show tunes—*Moon River, Jean, Born Free.* He even felt well enough to sing for a while. He had a beautiful voice; I hadn't heard him sing since the high school musicals.

The music and singing throughout our house warmed

away the chill of winter. As David sang and played, I felt grateful to participate in this moment with my folks. I was thankful that David was well enough that he could share his musical gift. It left a mark on us that time will never dim.

20

◆

*T*he winter became a memory, and spring—the spring of David's wish and desire—became reality. I found him outside by his flower bed, planting seeds. It had been months since he had ventured outdoors except to go to the doctors and the support group meetings. He was beaming as I crossed the yard to give him a hug.

"God heard me," he said brightly. "I made it to spring."

That he had. Packets of seeds lay atop the railroad ties, awaiting David's fingers to give them life.

He seemed dwarfed by the massive trees that lined his spacious back yard. He was a pale figure in contrast to the budding trees and returning greenery.

Although we continued the castor oil packs, the guided imagery, and creative visualizations, David was fading like a once-brilliant flower. I could see it and sense it. I accepted

the fact that he wasn't going to recover. The focus of the visualization sessions more and more became the light. I let
my imagination guide me as I led him through the sessions.
More frequently it was as if my intuition was saying, "Prepare him. Help him by letting him go." It was during this
time that I realized I couldn't give David the will to continue
to live in this world. I had often told him, "There are greater
worlds than this," and it became my focus to help prepare
him for those brighter, greater worlds.

For one day—the day he planted his seeds—it was a glorious moment in David's life. He had to be helped to the
chair by his garden, and his mother assisted him in the
planting, but for David it was the experience that he had
been heard: that God had answered his prayer to make it
through the winter.

The day he planted was not yet truly spring; its official
arrival was some weeks away. Winter, however, was merci-
ful in 1986. It seemed to me it had faded early so that David
could be outdoors in nature where he was at home. It is
unusual in Indiana for March to be anything but blustery
and cold. But in this year, spring came early; and I believe it
came for David, perhaps because the seasons knew he was
not long for this world.

I sat with David in the silence as he tended his garden.
The only conversation heard was between him and his future. Many people talk to their plants, but David spoke to
them before they were born. Perhaps that is why they flourished so.

That day was one of the last good days that David experienced.

Less than a week later, I received a frantic phone call from
Marianne. David had collapsed in his bedroom and was in-
coherent.

"David is not making sense," Marianne said. "He's in the
worst pain." I could hear the panic in her voice. She had

called the ambulance to take him to the emergency room. Luckily, they lived within two miles of the local hospital.

"Try to stay calm," I said, knowing it was a pointless remark to utter. "I'll meet you at the hospital."

"Please hurry," Marianne said.

In the back of my mind I knew that the hospital would eventually become a greater part of my time with David, and I dreaded it. There was an idealistic part of me that hoped that his music and gardening and painting would continue until he quietly and peacefully let go. In a sense I suppose I wanted to be spared being a part of David's agony, but that was not to be. I knew the reality of AIDS. I remembered all too well the nurse who referred to AIDS as "the monster." But I wanted to cling to the hope that maybe, maybe, David might go easily without the horrors that had ended so many other AIDS patients' lives. As I had been a part of the best of David's good days in the last months, I knew I would be a part of the worst of them as well. It left me with a feeling of sinking and dread. Not only for me, but for David and Marianne. The hardest part would be for Marianne. Losing a second son was still beyond my comprehension. I said a prayer for her.

I told my parents what was happening, grabbed my coat, and headed out the door. There was little traffic that night at 10:00 p.m. I arrived at the hospital parking lot fifteen minutes later. I parked the car and rushed through the emergency room doors.

Please, please, let it be easy on David. A prayer, a wish, a thought that was not to be granted—not that night.

There was a nurse behind the reception desk. I asked where David was.

"Are you a member of the family?" she asked, not looking up from her paperwork.

"Yes, I am."

"Go through those curtains, to your right."

I pushed through the curtained partitions that separated the patients and saw David lying on a cot. Marianne was holding his hand. Marianne's youngest daughter, Mary Jo, was standing on the other side of the cot, stroking David's head. Marianne had telephoned her right before she called me. David was in a fetal position, moaning. Marianne was frightened. I came over beside her.

"Where is that doctor?" she asked. Her eyes were bloodshot. She looked exhausted.

"The paramedics wheeled him in here without so much as an exam," Mary Jo said, disgusted. "They only checked his vital signs. We haven't seen a doctor or nurse yet." Mary Jo was twenty-three years old, pretty, brunette. She looked very much like Marianne. I had met her on several occasions. She was one of the family members outside of Lillian and Marianne who saw David often. She was—and had always been—fiercely protective of him.

I saw a nurse heading in the opposite direction, caught her attention, and rushed up to her.

"My friend over there is in a lot of pain," I said. "Can you give him a shot or something?" I had forgotten that only immediate family members were allowed to be with the patient in the emergency room.

"Is that your friend?" she asked, nodding toward David.

"Yes, it is," I said, confused by her tone of voice. It was cold.

"He'll have to wait a few minutes—we're busy at the moment." I looked around the emergency room and saw that very few of the partitions were closed. They weren't busy at all! The nurse's indifference angered me.

"Well, can you hurry up, please? He's in a lot of pain."

The nurse snapped at me. "*Your friend* is not the only patient we have here." I had to restrain myself from slapping her. Her voice dripped sarcasm on the words "your friend." I began to get the picture. She thought David was my companion or lover.

I pushed my rising anger aside and went back to Marianne, not repeating my dialogue with the nurse.

"I made him take a pain pill before we left," Marianne said, "but he threw up. It's never been this bad before." She was still holding David's hand, looking helpless and panicky.

"I just can't stand here while David suffers, Mom," Mary Jo said. "I'm going to get the doctor."

"Please don't say anything to upset them," Marianne pleaded, "or they won't help us at all."

"They're not helping us now," Mary Jo countered and disappeared between the curtains.

I knelt beside David. His face was ashen; dark circles like bruises surrounded his eyes. "It's going to be O.K., David," Marianne said, her voice quivering. "Hang on."

David was holding his stomach, moaning; his eyes clenched shut in pain. Beads of sweat stood out on his forehead. He wasn't talking at all. I began to say something to Marianne when Mary Jo's voice pierced through the emergency room.

"My brother is in *pain! Godammit! Somebody help him!*"

A young doctor with a clipboard appeared. Mary Jo was nearly pushing him through the partition. The physician looked barely old enough to have graduated from medical school.

He began to try to straighten David out of his fetal position. David nearly screamed. Marianne reacted with his pain and pleaded with the doctor. "Please give him something for the pain before you do anything."

The doctor was poker-faced and spoke in a monotone. "I need to find out what's wrong with him first."

"He's got AIDS," Mary Jo said loudly. "What else do you need to know?"

The young doctor looked around the emergency room self-consciously. He was irritated. "Would you mind keeping your voice down? I'm well aware he has AIDS. I want to see what's causing the acute pain."

Mary Jo sighed in disgust and shook her head. As Marianne recited the host of physical ailments David was suffering, Mary Jo and I exchanged unspoken thoughts:

He weighs less than ninety pounds and looks eighty years old. What else does the doctor need to know to give him the damn shot?

David's body was slowly and painfully shutting down. As was often the case, there was little treatment for the chronic pain of AIDS patients other than the administration of potent narcotic painkillers. I didn't have to be a physician to see that from David's physical condition he had only months to live—a year at best.

The physician tentatively probed David's abdomen and took his vital signs.

"Would you excuse me for a few minutes?" the doctor asked. "I want to examine him thoroughly." His tone of voice was indifferent and defensive.

He opened the curtain to let us out of the cubicle. Mary Jo didn't budge. "Mom, why don't you and Rob go have a cigarette." She looked at the doctor. "I'm staying. I'll let you know what's happening as soon as he's done." The doctor, thinking better of arguing, looked disgusted and said nothing.

Marianne nodded, and we went into the waiting room. We sat down and lit our cigarettes.

"Why is there always such a war with the medical people?" Marianne sighed and glanced at me through the cloud of smoke. "Would it be awful of me if I said I wished this were all over?" Tears ran from her eyes, and she dabbed them with a tissue. Marianne was a woman past the point of exhaustion. "I'm getting to the point where I can't stand to see him so uncomfortable."

I told her that her wish wasn't awful at all. David was getting worse and worse. "It would be easier if he would let go."

There, I had said it. Up to that point, I had been fearful to say those words. I was afraid of upsetting Marianne or perhaps I was afraid of my own guilt for feeling the meaning behind the words. I did want David to let go. I wanted it to be easy. I didn't want him to die a gruesome death.

"It's against nature," Marianne said, shaking her head. "It's against nature for a son to die before his parents. I went through this once and didn't think I'd live through it. And now—" her voice gave out, and her tears came freely—"and now . . . *this.*"

I felt helpless. What was there to say? I began to speak comforting words that sounded so empty—words that could not stave off Marianne's inner war, nor end the prospect of her losing her son.

Eventually she gave voice to her inner battle. "I think of needing to let David go, needing him to go on, and I think 'What kind of a mother are you?'" She shook her head, feeling the immensity of her guilt.

"I love David," Marianne said. "I love him more than my life. But *this,*" she gestured around the room. "I know it gets worse, and I'll be spending more time in hospitals. I know it gets more severe, and for his sake and my own I don't want it to. I don't think I can take it."

David was so lucky to have Marianne as a mother. I told her that she had endured so much and had been so strong. I also shared her thoughts.

"It's getting harder to see him like this," I added sympathetically. "I know he's going downhill, and I don't know what to do either." If anything, I wanted Marianne to know that she wasn't alone.

"It's strange," Marianne responded, "but I feel better just knowing that someone else feels a sense of what I do."

"I'll be here for you," I said.

We extinguished what was left of our cigarettes just as the

doctor came into the waiting room with Mary Jo following. Marianne and I stood up at the same time. The doctor's face was neutral. He showed neither compassion nor indifference. We were told that David was in critical need of a blood transfusion. The pain was being caused by his liver which was badly swollen, more so than usual. It was pressing against his other organs and causing severe cramping. The doctor said that he wanted to get a stool sample to check for internal bleeding.

"Did you give him a shot?" Marianne asked.

"I'll get the nurse to do that just as soon as I get —"

"No," Mary Jo interrupted. "The next thing you're going to do is give him the shot." She was standing close enough to the doctor to kiss him. "Morphine, heroin, I don't care—just don't allow him to suffer any more. *Now move!*"

Mary Jo was changing from anger to being emotionally upset. Her words to the doctor came out as a pathetic plea rather than a demand. The doctor had an expression of reluctance, as if morphine or Demerol® were in short supply. I wondered at his hesitancy. How was he able to examine David, see the pain, see the devastation of his condition, and be reluctant to relieve his pain?

"I'll see that he gets a shot immediately," he said, finally.

A nurse came over to administer the shot. David was still at the point where he couldn't speak, but he managed to whisper "Thank you" when she finished.

After a few minutes, he began to slowly uncurl. The Demerol® was mercifully beginning to take effect. He was, after twenty minutes, able to lie in a comfortable position.

The doctor returned with a specimen container so that David could give him a stool sample. He spoke with some hesitation.

"We have a slight problem," he said to Marianne. "We don't have a supply of your son's blood type here. We're having it sent from the Indiana University Medical Center in

Indianapolis. I'm afraid you're going to have to wait a couple of hours."

By this time it was after 11:00 p.m. By the time David would receive the transfusion, it would be after 2:00 a.m. when we got him home. Mary Jo was quick to offer a solution.

"Why don't you just admit David for the night?"

"There's no need for that," the doctor countered. "It's only a couple of hours until he'll be ready to go home."

Mary Jo spoke with strained patience. "My mother has to go to work at 5:00 a.m., Rob has to work in the morning, and so do I. There's no reason why you can't admit him for the night and we'll pick him up tomorrow."

"I can't do that," the doctor said.

"Why not?" the three of us asked simultaneously.

"Because there's no reason to," the doctor said again, adamantly.

Mary Jo's patience broke. "What do you mean there's no reason to? Look at my brother! He's very, very ill."

"I can see that," the doctor said wearily, "but there's nothing *chronically* wrong with him. I see that he's suffering from an ongoing debilitating illness. But all he needs is a transfusion."

"A transfusion that may not happen until 1:00 a.m.," Mary Jo said. "Doctor, are you short of beds in this hospital?"

The doctor looked at the floor, saying nothing. I couldn't believe it!

"No," the doctor sighed, "we don't have a shortage of beds. It's just —"

"Why don't you just say you don't want my brother in your hospital because he has AIDS?"

"That's not it at all," the doctor replied.

"Yes, that's exactly it," Mary Jo said. "Because he has AIDS, you're not going to admit him. You wouldn't let other people wait until 2:00 a.m. for a transfusion. You would admit them.

Now, I want you—"

A nurse came in and interrupted Mary Jo. "The blood will be here in thirty minutes," she said.

"Thank God," Marianne said. The doctor appeared immensely relieved.

"I want you to think about what you were asking us to do, doctor," Mary Jo said quietly. "I want you to remember that you would not admit a dying man to your hospital. I want you to think very long and very hard about that."

On that note, the doctor turned to walk away. "I'm sorry you feel that way, but that's not the case."

Marianne and Mary Jo stayed with David until the transfusion was complete, and they took him home. The stool sample revealed no internal bleeding. They put a castor oil pack on David's abdomen when he got home, and he slept through the night. A crisis had passed.

We had many miles to go, however, before we slept.

21

◆

I sat down with my journal one evening in April of 1986 and the entry turned into a letter to David:

Words I may say to David in time:

I'm here for you without condition. I know you understand I am not here to pity you, nor have I. But I am here to learn of you—and you me. The understanding of how we were brought together in this time is not in the design of material understanding. It is not by coincidence that we have met; for I have long since disbelieved in chance meetings. No, there is purpose here.

I need you to know that I am with you. I need you to know of the beliefs that have been distilled and have become a part of me since I have spent time with you: Your gifts, talents, creativity have taught me we are more than mere mortals. We are some sort of divine instruments of a power or force that goes beyond the dogmatic, traditional sketches of what humanity calls God. I believe us to be aspects of that One Creative Force. How else can the beauty of art and nature and music be explained? The majestic designs of this Force play through us again and again—no matter what state we find ourselves in. You, in your dying, are a vibrant picture of the living—the living we are supposed to be about: relishing each day, savoring each moment, not forgetting the beauty around us. Divine? Yes. Inspired? Indeed. Simple? Of course. I think, most of all, that is one of the greatest discoveries I have found with you. That the truly divine is truly simple.

The creativity we find in the moment goes on with us—for we are, in a divine sense, a magical moment of God, happening briefly on earth to magnify the Creator's capability to express Itself. These are things that have been awakened in me. If I had to wager all I had, all that I am, it would be on the idea that we are beings that far transcend this body—which is at times such a hindrance to the soul. We also transcend time and space and anything limited. Our bodies are not where we began, nor where we will end, it is merely our current residence for a brief shining moment in a material world.

If it is true that you find your time in this lifetime to be short, in this body that has become painful baggage, know that you are on the threshold of a new beginning. Death in the physical world is but a birth into the spiritual world. You are near that spiritual birth. You are in the midst of a transition that you must pass through before that glorious spiritual birth. And after you make that transition back to where you came from, I will be with you in spirit. I will be here for you now and in the future. I will be here to help you through this as physically as I can, and I will be there as spiritually as I can when you leave the body behind.

Things are hard right now—but I know the understanding will come. Even as you have given me understanding that life and death are but shades and shadows in one long continuous experience, you will gain understanding when you leave this realm behind. Remember the light we so often see and speak of in the meditations. It will be your guide and guardian. Remember that all you are in spirit is timeless and ageless. Nothing is lost. I believe with all my heart these things are true. You are an inspiration to me, and this is not good-by. Remember me when you face the dawn in your new world. I love you."

My journal was a place of solace for me during David's difficult days. There were few people I could talk with about him, outside of the support group, my parents, and David's family. Much of the experiences I had gone through I kept to myself and wrote down in my journal.

There was one friend of mine I had been in contact with since high school who was a sounding board to my experiences with David. Darrell Cook and I had performed in many plays together in high school. We had been in several musicals with David. He had not seen David since the high school days. David frequently asked about our mutual friends; few of his one-time friends saw him in his last months.

David looked forward to seeing old friends again. The isolation was the hardest part of his illness. He was very outgoing and social. The loneliness was overwhelming for him. At a time when I mentioned Darrell, David asked me to bring him to his home.

Darrell and I went one evening. As we entered the house, David was playing at the piano. We stood and listened for several minutes. He never sounded better, I thought.

I tried as well as I could to prepare Darrell for David's condition. Although he greeted David warmly and hugged him, the shock at his deterioration registered in his eyes. Nevertheless, Darrell remembered that David was still very much an old friend, and we had a wonderful evening together. David continued to play his music for Darrell and me.

As the night wound to a close, David become philosophical, and we had one of our deepest conversations about the nature of life and death.

"I just wonder what it's all for," David said to Darrell and me. "I mean the purpose of life—why we're here."

I launched into what I had learned from my reading of people's near-death experiences. The majority of those who had glimpsed the after-death state returned with a renewed enthusiasm for living life to the fullest. But above all else, they said that learning to love was the most important thing.

"So many people said they saw their entire lives before them," I said. "Every thought and deed of their lifetime was portrayed in this panoramic view, all at once."

I explained one case in which a Being of Light asked a person in this after-death place, "What did you do with your life?"

"Wow!" David exclaimed. "That's heavy. It's like a judgment? Like the Bible said?"

"Sort of," I replied. "More, the person realized that this Being of Light wasn't asking so much, 'What did you do with your life?' in terms of deeds, but in a sense of 'How did you live your life in terms of love? Did you learn love?' The people who had this experience said that everything they thought was important was now meaningless if it wasn't based on unconditional love. The purpose of life, many of them concluded, was that life is giving us the opportunity to learn love."

I told them about George Ritchie, the physician who had been clinically dead for nine minutes. He had said that this Being of Light loved him beyond measure; there was no condemnation or judgment in this light. Rather it was he who had to judge his life on the measure of how well he learned the lesson of love. The physician eventually wrote the book, *Return from Tomorrow,* which detailed his death experience.

"But," I explained, "these people said they never felt more awake, more alive in their whole lives as they did in this 'death' experience."

"And learning love was the most important thing," David repeated tentatively.

"It makes sense," Darrell said, "when you think that the Bible said that 'God is love, and love is God.' If that is what God is, then that is what we're supposed to manifest."

David pondered. It was as if he were coming to some major understanding. "And when we learn love—in our own way—then our mission is complete here on earth?"

Darrell and I agreed that yes, when we learn what we came to learn, then we pass on.

David nodded. He was in a silent space, very contemplative. The hour was getting late, and Darrell and I said our good-bys.

Darrell was upset during the drive home. "I kept thinking about us on stage. Looking at David, I got the feeling that our days of high school seemed like a century ago, yet I know it was only a few years."

We talked about David's music. Darrell was as moved by it as I. "How can he play like that when he can barely walk?" Darrell asked. "It gave me chills."

I related what I had learned since meeting David: Sometimes there are compensations. David was dying, yes. But it was during the process of dying that he was very, very close to the Divine. It enabled him to express that divinity in his music.

"It was like listening to something godlike," Darrell said.

I didn't understand the whole of the issue of AIDS, but being around David helped me understand that there was indeed something that was continuing to say, "All is well. I know how it looks, but all really is well."

22

The day after Darrell and I had visited David, Marianne called.

"I need you again, Rob," Marianne said. "David has taken an overdose. He's unconscious." Her voice sounded too even, too calm. She might have been in shock.

"A deliberate overdose or an accident?"

"Deliberate."

"I'm on my way," I said, not asking her to explain.

Suicide? David?

David had not been his usual self the night before. I couldn't put my finger on what was different about him.

Resolved?

Yes, there was a sense of resolve about him. A kind of determined acceptance—if there was such a thing. David asked Darrell and me so many questions. He asked all the

177

things I had wanted to talk to him about—the purpose of life, why we're here . . .

He asked all those questions as if he were making some sort of major decision.

I was trying to piece it all together without knowing the circumstances of his overdose. Maybe it was accidental and Marianne was mistaken. My thoughts were in a whirlwind as I sped through town heading for David's house. I said a prayer and asked for guidance.

Marianne was at the front door when I drove up to the house. I ran the length of the sidewalk up the front steps. She opened the door for me.

"I haven't moved him," she said. "I haven't called anybody except you."

Marianne hadn't been crying. She was wide-eyed. *Shell-shocked*, I thought. We rushed into David's room. He was sitting at his desk where he did most of his drawing and painting. He was face down on the desk. Empty pill bottles lay everywhere. Blood was all over him and the desk. I had to tell myself repeatedly to stay calm.

I grabbed his left arm and checked his pulse. His skin was cool; his pulse was faint and rapid. My mind tried to take in what I was seeing, but wasn't doing a very good job of it.

That's not blood. It's paint. David had gotten paint all over him. Small oil paint containers were open and spilled.

After I made sure that David's heart was beating and that he was breathing, even though it was shallow, I began to move him.

"I saw David before I went to bed," Marianne said. "Around midnight. He said he was going to paint for a while and could put himself to bed. I left him! Rob, I should have—"

"Help me get him up," I said. "Let's get him to the bed."

David resembled a clown with a bad make-up job. The situation would have been comical had he merely passed out. The horror of the situation hit me full force when I looked down at the canvas David was painting. It was smeared, but its message struck me like a slap in the face. Words were written with a framed, flowered border; a very creative suicide note. He'd obviously lost consciousness before he finished the gilded edges of the painting.

"I learned how to love," the painting read. The meaning of the words came crashing home. The previous night's conversation, the questions, David's contemplative state, the empty bottles lying everywhere; this was David's "exit"— this was his suicide note.

Oh, dear God, that's not what I meant! That's not what I meant at all!

I was nearly hysterical as we moved David to the bed. I was in tears, and my hands were shaking; I again checked his vital signs. His heartbeat was faint but steady. His breathing was labored.

I quickly explained to Marianne the conversation that David, Darrell, and I had had. "I told him that when we learn how to love, our mission in this lifetime is over." I remarked to her that this was my fault. It was as if the worst possible happening had come out of what was a thoughtful conversation.

This time it was Marianne who came to my emotional rescue. "This is not your fault," she barked. "This is David's fault. Stop that."

All of this had happened in just a matter of a few minutes. The situation had the slow, running-through-molasses quality of a nightmare. Marianne's quick response to my panic brought me back to a calmer sense of reality. We looked at the empty pill bottles. There were so many. Lorazepam®, Tylenol® with codeine, dilaudid, Compazine®, Reglan®.

They're all depressants. He's taken enough pills to kill a horse.

"How's his breathing?" Marianne asked.

"Steady. But I don't know how," I said, looking at all the

pill bottles. I knelt beside the bed and called out David's name several times loudly, waiting for a response. There was none. I pinched the skin on his forearm. Still no response.

"I tried to rouse him before you got here," Marianne said. "Nothing. He didn't flinch."

There was blood on his abdomen, not paint. I lifted his shirt, and there was a horizontal slash across his stomach, oozing blood. At first I thought he had cut himself, then I realized that David had slumped at the desk all night after he passed out. The rough edge of the wooden desk had cut into his stomach.

Hours—he lay like this for hours. Marianne had checked on him just after midnight; it was now 10:00 o'clock in the morning. I estimated that he was unconscious at his desk for at least eight hours.

"Jesus, what a mess!" I went into the kitchen to call Dan, the physician in charge of the support group. I didn't know whether we should take him to the hospital, call an ambulance, give him black coffee—I was clueless. Dan finally answered the phone, and I quickly explained the situation, listing the empty drug bottles I found around him. Dan instructed me to count David's pulse and his breathing rate per minute and report back to him. I went into the bedroom where Marianne was attempting to clean the paint off his face. David lay motionless. Marianne's face was nearly expressionless as I took his pulse and counted his breaths.

"How could he do this to me?" Marianne hissed. "After all the weeks and months—*the years*—I've been here for him. Now this. Not a note, a thank you, an 'I'm sorry.' Just this mess." I mistook Marianne's calm for shock. It wasn't shock; she was angry. Furious.

I went back to the phone and gave Dan the vitals.

"Don't ask me how it's possible," Dan said with a sigh, "but David is going to live. His vitals are very strong considering all the drugs he took. He'll probably be unconscious for the next two days, but he's going to make it. I'd advise you to send him to I.U. Med Center so that they can monitor him. They'll also want to pump his stomach." I covered the mouthpiece momentarily:

"David's going to make it," I said loudly so that Marianne could hear me from the kitchen.

I asked Dan if there was anything more we should do. We were to watch him until the medical team arrived and make sure to keep him turned on his side in case he vomited. Dan said he probably didn't vomit because of the Compazine® and Reglan®, both antinauseant drugs. He also told me to bag all the empty bottles so that the paramedics would know what David had taken.

"Half of a pharmacy," I said, amazed at the array of pills David had consumed and yet still lived.

"It's amazing," Dan said. "The amount of drugs he took would have killed anyone else. Very strange."

"Around David," I said in agreement, "I've gotten used to the unusual."

Dan asked me if I was coming to the support group the next night. I usually came with David. He wasn't going to be in any shape to go anywhere other than a hospital. I decided to go alone. For once, I needed to go alone.

"Yes, I'll be there." I thanked Dan and hung up the phone. Marianne was rinsing out the washcloth in the sink. Paint colors swirled down the drain.

"I can't believe David has left me with this mess," Marianne said again. She was angry, but close to tears. I'd never seen her angry at David before. "He'd have seen fit to die like that," she said. I remembered Marianne was Catholic, so this incident hit her doubly hard.

"What didn't I do?" she asked no one in particular. "What didn't I do to keep him comfortable? After all of this time, this is what it comes down to? I just can't believe it."

This time I spoke and repeated the words she'd spoken to

me, that this was David's doing. It was a feeble attempt to make her feel better. We both were feeling undone, guilty.

I followed her into his room as she continued to clean David. The guilt hit me again full force. Where had I failed? What had I not done? As I stood asking myself questions that there were no answers to at the moment, my own guilt was turning into anger. Finally all I could feel was sadness.

I failed him. I felt such despair.

As the scenario turned over and over in my mind, I tried to see it from David's perspective. He's been in excruciating pain and miserable. He was lonely. Yes, he's to the point where I could understand if he wanted help in ending this life, ending this condition he's afflicted with. What upset me immensely was the fact that he would have left us forever wondering, "Did I do enough? Was it something I didn't say that could have prevented his suicide?" It was the fact that he would have left us with the guilt. For Marianne, in a lot of ways, it was the ultimate slap in the face. A death without closure, without a good-by.

Perhaps the divine forces that run this universe had said, "No, David. You're not making this transition like this. You have things yet to do and say."

Marianne called Mary Jo and she came over. Marianne was still cleaning up David when Mary Jo made the call to the paramedics.

"Why didn't you two call an ambulance?" Mary Jo asked.

Marianne and I stood and looked at each other, our expressions blank. In all the chaos and confusion, we hadn't called the ambulance. I felt as if I were coming unhinged. Mary Jo's question remained unanswered.

Once I had found David breathing and stable, I had turned within, wondering about my role in David's suicide attempt. I wasn't thinking clearly. How can you possibly think straight under these circumstances?

Mary Jo was devastated by David's attempt. She felt the

same loss that Marianne and I did, that David would have "left without saying good-by." That aspect, the bottom line of this whole scene, didn't set well with any of us. A depressive cloud had settled over the house.

The Morgan paramedics were quick to respond, arriving in less than ten minutes. One of them was trying to rouse David by slapping his face and talking loudly in his ear.

A young paramedic, she looked to be about twenty, gathered up the pill bottles.

"Jesus," she said, reading the drug labels. She looked at the rescue team in amazement. "And he's still breathing!"

As the paramedics loaded David onto the stretcher, Mary Jo, Marianne, and I stood by and silently watched. David was to be taken to Indiana University Medical Center in Indianapolis. Mary Jo suggested one or all of us follow the ambulance.

"He's going to be unconscious for a while," the paramedic said. She must have seen the fatigue on our faces. "Why don't you plan on coming up tomorrow. They'll keep him for observation for several days at least. Given his condition and the suicide attempt, he'll probably be in the hospital for a while."

Marianne and I put our arms around each other, feeling weary beyond words. She looked as if she hadn't slept in days. There was, however, a sense of relief on seeing David loaded into the ambulance. We decided to let the paramedics go without us.

It was too early in the day for a beer, even though a cold one sounded wonderful after all this. We sat down for coffee instead.

As the ambulance sped away, the siren's wail gradually faded until the morning stillness returned. I told Marianne about the previous night, the conversations, David's strange behavior. Marianne sipped her coffee and was surprisingly composed.

"I know I'm not the most devout Catholic," she said, "but David knows how I feel about suicide. He knows. Lately he's been talking about what a burden he's been and how sorry he is for all of this. I should have seen it coming. I just didn't."

"Neither did I," I said. The scene of David lying in the paint replayed over and over in my mind. The painting itself haunted me.

"Marianne, when I told David that I felt our purpose was to learn how to love—I didn't know he was searching for a rationale for suicide."

"I know that. This was no one's fault. I have to keep telling myself that." She shook her head. "God, but people feel so responsible when someone tries suicide or succeeds at it. Always wondering, 'What could I have done?' That's what makes me angry, Rob."

I tried to put myself in David's shoes. I wondered if I would have lived as long or endured as much as he had. It wasn't really that far-fetched that he would attempt suicide. What was far-fetched was the absence of a note, a letter— something. David was a caring person, always conscious of the feelings of other people. But not this time. The logical voice of my intuition told me the story: David had reached the point where he couldn't walk without assistance. He had lost control of his independent life. He was in pain most of the time. How frustrating that must be for a former athlete! Yes, I could understand why he did it.

But why didn't he succeed? Why did he not die?

Marianne speculated and I agreed. "Because, whatever God has planned for David, this wasn't the time for his 'arrival' over there. It just plain wasn't his time."

We sat in silence at the kitchen table, the noonday sun pouring through the kitchen window. The bright sunny day seemed so out of context from the morning's events. It should have been raining, cloudy.

I told Marianne of an Edgar Cayce reading I had read

some years before in which suicide was discussed. Cayce's view was that no one is an island, that we do not live only for ourselves. He reminded his questioner that part of our mission is to help others. If we commit suicide, we're not only depriving ourselves, but also causing pain in other people. But David felt that he was causing immense pain in other people. He felt like an incredible burden. In many ways, I guess he thought this would end the suffering for all concerned. In one way, it would; but in another way, people would forever feel responsible.

Marianne said she realized why there was no noticeable signs that precipitated the suicide attempt: If there were and we sensed it coming, one of us would have talked him out of it.

I disagreed. If David had come to me and said, "I'm really suffering and miserable. I want help in dying. I want you and my mom to be there, but I want to let go. This is too much. Please help me," I probably would have helped him.

But Marianne and I differed. I could see her point. "In what David just attempted," Marianne said, "there're no good-bys—there's nothing left." I agreed with her. There was no closure. We had all been through so much together for it to end this way. I found myself vacillating among anger, guilt, and sadness. Of the three, sadness was the greatest. All of this was very sad indeed. David must have felt so alone and so afraid.

Marianne said that she would go to Indianapolis later that evening. For the rest of the day she was going to rest. I got up to leave, hugged her, and promised to visit David the following day. She said she'd telephone me after her visit.

"You're one of the family," she said, as I was going out the door. "You know that, don't you? We couldn't have made it this far without you."

I hugged her again and realized one of those intangible rewards that come along with what I had committed myself to. It was one of the rewards the social worker had spoken of at the training seminar: I never felt closer to a human being in my entire life than I did at that moment with Marianne. It was a tragic, terrible moment. But at the same time it was vital, meaningful; it was *life*. We felt the calm in the midst of the storm, and I was grateful for it.

———

David was awake, groggy, and unhappy in I.U. Medical Center. His stomach had been pumped; they had administered drugs to reverse the depressive effects of the narcotics, and he was given replenishing I.V. fluids. They found high levels of all the drugs he took in his bloodstream. He was considered something of a "miracle" case by the hospital. Dilaudid is a potent narcotic painkiller, and the dose David had taken of the drug would have killed the average person. Dilaudid depresses the central nervous system, and the body stops breathing. David, however, never stopped breathing.

When Marianne telephoned, she said that David was very angry, thinking that "heroic" measures were used to save him. Again, I tried to understand why it hadn't been time for David to die. A lesson I learned about AIDS is that the body can take a whole lot in the way of dreadful illnesses and yet keep living. David's situation was even more amazing because physically there wasn't much left of him at that point. He was literally beginning to resemble a human skeleton. But his spirit was another matter. It was fiery and vibrant. I had a feeling it would be right to the end.

"Brace yourself," Marianne said. "David is not a happy camper. They're going to keep him for a while."

But David had awakened more than angry; he was furious. He had taken an arsenal of drugs to end his nightmare; yet he had awakened and the nightmare continued.

The following evening I drove to the medical center. I walked into his private room.

"Thank you very much," he said curtly, as I walked into the room. David was very much awake—and mad as hell. "Thank you for bringing me back to *this*," he gestured around the room.

"I didn't bring you back, Dave," I said, equally short. "God or somebody brought you back. It wasn't time for you to go. And damn it! Don't you dare speak to me like that." David was caught off guard momentarily. He'd never seen me angry. He was sitting up in his hospital bed, shaking his head back and forth, blaming me for his survival.

"You called the paramedics; they resuscitated me. They had to."

I began pacing his room, feeling the anger rising within me, feeling as though David had simply decided to die and to hell with everyone else. I let him have it.

"How do you think it made me feel to find you lying in that painting?" I was forceful and upset. David wouldn't meet my gaze.

" 'I learned how to love.' Christ, that was too perfect, David. You ask me about the meaning of life and then pull the plug, without so much as leaving a note." David was looking out the window. A magazine, open and unread, lay in his lap. I forced myself to be calm.

"I felt responsible. Your mom did, too. We felt as if we both failed."

David was seething with anger, but underneath it I saw a hurt child, who merely wanted to end the pain.

"You don't understand," David said in an even tone. "You don't understand at all."

"Talk to me," I pleaded.

The last two years of the horror David had endured came pouring out, a flood of misery, loneliness, and pain. His eyes were haunted and tired.

"Mom is exhausted. I can see you're exhausted, too. I'm at the point where I can't make it to the bathroom on my

own any more. The other day I didn't make it. I messed myself just like a child." David raised his voice in a frustration
so futile that it quenched my anger and brought tears to my
eyes. He was on the verge of tears himself.

"*You have no idea what this is like. This is hell.*"

The nurse momentarily stuck her head in the door and
asked if everything was all right. I mumbled something that
everything was fine, when it was not. I lit a cigarette.

"Yes, I thought suicide was the answer," David explained.
"I thought it would all be over. Over. Don't you see that I
wanted it to be easier than just wasting away? I wanted to
end Mom's worrying. She worries about me, and I can't
stand it." David's tears came out freely. It was a rare occasion when he cried. I went over and sat with him on the bed.

"God let me see the spring," David said, sobbing. "I
thought it was enough. I thought it was a sign that it was
O.K. to leave now. I thought it would be better for everybody."

"I wish you had told me," I said. "David, nobody did anything to bring you back. No resuscitation attempts; nothing.
You never stopped breathing." I gave him a blow-by-blow
description of the morning that we found him.

"You survived on your own," I said, finishing the story.

"For Christ's sake, why?" he asked, exasperated, tearful.
"Rob, I can't walk any more, I'm throwing up blood, I can't
eat. What is left for me to do?"

It was one of those moments in which I wished I could
pull a book off the shelf and give the needed answer. I
couldn't.

"I don't know," I said finally. "But, David, your Mom and I
are in this with you, too. You are my friend. If you had died
like that I don't know what I would have done."

David began to protest, saying that it had nothing to do
with me; for the first time he said that I had helped him immensely. I asked him to put himself in my place. How would

he have felt if a friend committed suicide? David was silent for a moment, then with tears in his eyes said, "I'd have felt like you do. I'm sorry, Rob." Tears rolled down his cheeks.

"Your mother needs to know that she did everything she could to help you," I said. "A suicide would tell her she failed."

David confessed that he genuinely thought his death would bring a quietude to our lives. He thought it would end the sadness, the tragedy, and the dependency.

"When I look in the mirror," he added, "I don't see me any more. I see AIDS, and I think—'How can anybody put up with this?'" David was bewildered and horrified at what he had physically become. When he looked in the mirror, he saw a monster. He thought everyone saw the same thing. We didn't. We saw the essence of David. It was a revelation to him to hear that, yes, beyond the emaciation and the physical illnesses that plagued him we still loved him.

"Really?" he asked, genuinely surprised.

"Really," I answered.

I told him that maybe he had one more musical piece to compose; perhaps he was to stay around to see his flowers bloom. Finally I said that perhaps "they" weren't ready yet to have him be "born" onto the other side.

"Obviously they don't want me yet," he said with a hint of sarcasm. "Maybe my 'suite' isn't ready."

Just as David was beginning to lighten up and laugh, a coughing fit seized him. I grabbed the basin and held it for him as he coughed up blood and mucus. It went on for minutes that felt like hours. Again, all I could do was place my hand on his shoulder and hold the basin as he coughed and vomited. Eventually he stopped, and I helped him lie back on the bed as he wept and asked me, "When, Rob? When will it be over?"

I was overcome with that futile sense of helplessness. I just held him as he cried.

Dear God, please, help him. Help me help him.

23

◆

*D*avid stayed in the hospital for several weeks. The care he received was the complete opposite of his earlier trip to the emergency room. The staff at Indiana University Medical Center were wonderful and sympathetic, and the nursing staff genuinely liked David. Knowing he was in good medical hands gave me a break. Marianne made the drive to Indianapolis to see him every day. I didn't, and I tried my best not to feel guilty about it. So much had happened in David's life—and my own—in the past few months that I needed some days to myself.

My parents were understanding during this period. The crises in which I had passed with David brought me closer to them. They became like soul-companions, and we often talked of metaphysical subjects. Mom spoke more about her own near-death occurrence. Part of the experience that she carried from that brief encounter was the certainty that death was by no means "the end." Hearing her talk of this gave me comfort. We were never a religious family, yet we each had deeply meaningful spiritual values. My time with David enabled us to share those values as a family. Dad and I had deep discussions about Edgar Cayce, and I shared the conversations I had had with Hugh Lynn. I even told them of my own near-death experience.

Some of our family's relatives were disparaging because my parents didn't raise their children to go to church. I was especially thankful that they did not. It enabled me to pursue spirituality on my own. Our family became religiously diverse, but extremely open to the varieties of religious thought. Jim, my middle brother, became a Catholic; my oldest brother, John, maintained his own belief in Christianity very much like my parents, yet wasn't dogmatic. We were very "free-spirited" in a religious sense, and it made our lives richer when we discussed and shared our different views of God, life, death, and the hereafter.

When my folks asked me about David, I admitted I had reached the point where I understood a passage in the Cayce readings which pointed out that sometimes death is a healing. It was going to be a relief when he let go. I didn't feel badly about this. In my mind's eye, I knew David to be in the throes of a great transition from death to life. His passage would be a relief.

Several days before he came home from the hospital, I ventured to the woods that had been my refuge in my early life. The trails were overgrown a bit, but still passable. I made my way over the hills and through gullies, listening to the unchangeable voices of nature. I sat near the old beech tree and quietly meditated. It was calmer than calm, as if the recent turbulent days made this period of quiet, quieter still. I said a prayer of thanks for it all and hoped I had done and said the right things.

My field of vision became illuminated while meditating. It began as a light that merely became brighter. Then, the light became a profile of Jesus. Windswept hair, dark piercing eyes, and a smile. It was as if His face had always been in this background of my meditations—rather like looking at a three-dimensional puzzle when the picture is so clear that it cannot be seen. When I realized I was seeing the face of Christ, He turned, looked directly at me—smiling—and the image faded from view, leaving the white background.

It sounds incredulous, yet at the time of this vision, it was the most ordinary experience in God's natural setting of the woods. It left me feeling that I had been heard, much in the same way I had been heard in the past. A divine acknowledgment.

There had indeed been the storm, but I found the calm, even as He promised.

"Be with David," I said aloud to the fading vision. "Help him over this last hurdle." Nature—one of the many voices of God—answered in the winds and sky and woods as it did years before: "I am with you always, even unto the end."

I arose from my meditation, stretched, breathed in the springtime air and sun, and made my way home, remembering a passage from the Cayce readings, that whoever understands nature walks close with God. It wasn't a concept at all; it was right here.

———

When I next spoke with Marianne, she said that David had talked to her about the suicide attempt. He had cried for several days after his angry visit with me and had apologized to her for what he had done.

"I told David what I've said all along," Marianne said. "He's not a burden, he's my son." She also told him that she loved him now just as much as she ever did.

David came home. It became obvious, after he was home

two weeks, that he had reached the point where he needed twenty-four-hour-a-day care. The painkillers weren't working well any more.

By the first of May, little more than a month after his suicide attempt, what remained of David's health had rapidly deteriorated. He could only digest protein drinks and milkshakes and could barely keep those on his stomach. He couldn't sleep for long intervals; the fevers were raging and keeping him in a near delirious state. His bedroom was on the opposite side of the house from Marianne's. She moved him into the spare bedroom next to hers so that she could hear him when he called.

She made arrangements to have David admitted to the hospice care center in Indianapolis. She had frequently told him that she would take care of him as long as she was physically able. If conditions reached the stage where he required around-the-clock care, as he did now, they had agreed that a hospice center was the best place for him. The hospital staff had wanted to admit him to the hospice center after his suicide attempt, but David had chosen to go home and Marianne honored his decision. It was only for a short while, however. Lillian was worried about something happening during the time that Marianne and I were at work. David's mind had begun to be affected after he returned home. He had moments when he was delirious, talking incoherently. Most of the time, though, he was clear and lucid in his thinking. Then there would be lapses. He also developed a tendency to lose his balance and fall. Because of her age and her arthritis, Lillian wasn't able to help David to his feet, and he couldn't get up by himself. A hospice center would provide a quiet, caring atmosphere during his final weeks or months.

Before he was taken to the hospice center, however, David asked us to help him outside so that he could see his roses and spring flowers. Marianne and I both helped him walk to the side yard, where his beautiful roses were flourishing in the springtime sun. David caressed the red petals and talked quietly to them as he always did with his plants.

Another answered prayer, I thought. *Thank you for letting David see his roses in bloom.*

"The roses sure are pretty this year, Mom."

"They sure are, David."

His spring flowers had also come up and were blooming. Because he was so weak during the planting, he had scattered the seeds haphazardly and the flowers came up in a hodgepodge bush-like fashion. It made a wild, colorful arrangement in the corner of the yard.

"That is totally out of hand," David said chuckling, pointing to the disarrayed flowers, "but it was the best I could do. I'm just glad they're blooming."

"It looks like a Monet," I said.

"They look confused," David corrected. "Sorry, guys," he said to the flowers, laughing. As Marianne and I stood on either side of David, walking him around the yard, we shared the feeling that this was the last time David would see his flowers. Marianne had been so strong for David and, even at this knowing, she smiled at me. In her eyes I saw strength and power beyond my understanding. She had said many times that it was God who had enabled her to get up in the morning and be about her work. Even so, I never ceased to be amazed at the resiliency of the soul. I loved Marianne.

David was drowsy from the narcotics, the dose of which had to be doubled since he had returned from the hospital. Marianne had begun to administer David's medicines when he needed them. She kept them well out of his reach.

We finally helped David into the house, assuming he would be ready to lie down. He wasn't. "To the piano," he ordered. We carefully guided him into the living room to the piano bench and put the pillow down for him to sit upon.

He didn't have the strength to open the wooden fallboard that covered the piano keys. We opened it for him. David sighed as he looked at the keys, his hands—so thin that I could see his pulse on his wrist—were poised above the keys. Marianne and I stood by him. Lillian was in her favorite chair. David was hesitant, looking frightened, almost as if he were saying, "What if I can't?"

"You can do it, honey," Lillian said. "Go on."

David looked at each of us, closed his eyes, and began to play. Haltingly at first, then the music smoothed out. It was rough going, but there were—as usual—the magical movements that sent chills through us all. I don't think there was a dry eye when he completed his improvisational piece. He smiled and asked us to help him back to bed. He slowly but surely was saying his "good-bys" to everything: his gardens, music, and—in his own way—to us. There was a sense of peace about the house and about David. When we finally took him back to bed, he was almost instantly asleep.

————

Several days before Marianne took David to the hospice center, his mind started to wander and grow foggy. He began to forget day-to-day events, and people were becoming vague to him. Though I'd seen him the day before, he asked me why it had been so long since I had last seen him. By the time he was checked into St. Vincent's Hospice Care Center in Indianapolis, he was in and out of consciousness most of the time.

Marianne had some emotional difficulty checking him into the center. Not because of the workers, but because she knew her son would spend his remaining days there. The nursing staff sat down with her, gave her a glass of wine, and talked about the hospice program. They gave her a hug as she left the center.

"Rob, they are wonderful," Marianne said. "So caring. It's

not like a hospital at all. David has his own room, and they said we can fill it with his personal items."

I was not surprised; hospice care centers were started by Elisabeth Kübler-Ross some twenty years earlier. The purpose of hospice was to care for individuals who had six months or less to live. The nursing staff was trained to keep the patients as comfortable as possible and maintain as much of a "home-away-from-home environment" as possible. There was a music room, a small library, and a sun room. The workers at St. Vincent's established a first-name relationship with Marianne, always greeted her warmly, and offered to help her in any way they could.

The day I visited David at the center, Marianne introduced me to the nurses and I was given a tour of the facilities. I was treated like a member of the family. David's room was very near the nurse's station. He was sleeping when I entered his room with Marianne. We both sat in the silence, feeling a sense of peace. The only sound in the room was David's labored breathing. Marianne then stood beside David's bed and caressed his hair.

"He's had a long, hard road," she said. "I think he's almost home now." David didn't stir.

Maybe it was the seeming finality of it all, the feeling that David's passing was inevitable, knowing that the crises had drawn us all closer together. I cried. There was no feeling of loss, only a cleansing. Marianne walked me outside David's room. We decided to take the nurse's offer of a glass of wine.

Sitting in the sun room, Marianne told me that her sister-in-law, Gayle, had died the night before. I was in shock. That vibrant creature I had met six months before was gone?

Marianne told me that she had gone downhill swiftly and had died at home in Florida with her family by her side. The doctors had been right in their prognosis. At the time I had met Gayle, the cancer had spread throughout most of her body. The brief visit I had with her replayed in my mind. In that short meeting, I saw a light aglow within her, a light that delighted in the fun, frolic, and *living* of life. She had crossed my mind over the last few months, and Marianne had kept me abreast of her condition. For some reason, I always thought that David would die before Gayle. So did Marianne. Mainly because Gayle was so outgoing and vivacious last winter. Yet, the cancer seized her with the swiftness of a summer storm and left her just as quickly. She didn't survive that storm, but for the time she was alive, she lived to the fullest. She set up trust funds for her children and personally took care of her business affairs. She didn't seem to spend any time being fearful or in a state of denial; she quietly and quickly got her affairs in order and prepared for her "departure" as one would prepare for a trip abroad. There was something courageous about Gayle, and I never forgot her.

Again it was like seeing that candle that burns brightest before burning out.

Sitting in the hospice center, I thought of Gayle and David and remembered a quote from hospice founder, Elisabeth Kübler-Ross:

> "People are like stained-glass windows. The true beauty can be seen only when there is light from within. The darker the night, the brighter the windows."

24

◆

*D*avid was anxious. "I feel as if there's something left for me to do." He was dozing in and out of a morphine haze, but was still coherent. "I feel as if I'm supposed to do something."

I was sitting next to David's bed, holding his hand. "David, maybe you just need to let go." Those words didn't come easily. The sound of them to my own ears seemed foreign, heavy. David was near death. This time, there would be no reprieve, no medical intervention—there was no more time. Looking at him was like gazing upon the fading light of a candle. His passage was imminent.

David is dying.

Yes. A part of me was *feeling* David's passing as well as being a witness to it. As much as I had been through with him, I could literally feel that his dying was the preparation for him to be born into a new life, a new world. Being near him now, I knew his unusual consciousness would go on, survive, prosper. These thoughts lent a certain calmness, a peace to our last minutes together.

David looked up at me, and he looked so *old*. Not just because of the lines of his face and his wasted body. But his eyes reflected a lifetime of experiences. I was grateful to see David was without fear.

"Do you think it would be all right?" David asked. "To let go, I mean."

Would it be all right? I thought of the pain, the ravages of AIDS that David had endured. I remembered Cayce saying that many things in life were more difficult than making the transition at death. Even so, I knew I would miss David—he had become a dear friend. But, oh, to shed that body, to be free!

Finally feeling a breakthrough of emotion through the tears, I found myself smiling. "Yeah, Dave, I think it would be O.K. You have, as they say, 'fought the good fight.' I've learned so much from you."

He came out of his dozing and appeared puzzled. "What could you possibly have learned from me?" There was a tone of dismissal in his voice.

I explained to him the courage he showed in facing life with AIDS. David was an example of someone who had learned to live with it—creatively. I reminded him of his music and his art.

"I'm glad you liked it, Rob. I loved playing before an 'audience' besides my family." He smiled his smile at me. His eyes were drowsy, far away, contented. "And you know I've always been such a ham." I nodded in agreement, both of us laughing. A nurse came in chatting away about how good it was to hear laughter. She unlocked a cabinet next to David's bed and opened a small vial of oral solution morphine.

"Better than bourbon," David said to the nurse. "You

know, if you bottled this stuff and sold it, the world would be much more pleasant." The nurse was nodding her head in earnest. I couldn't help from laughing. *Exit laughing*, I thought. *Why not?*

The nurse fussed over David, fixing his pillows, mothering him. When she left, David lay back on the bed.

"Would you lead me through one of the meditations before you go?" David asked. "I think I need it."

"Of course. My pleasure," I said. "But first I want to read you something."

I had brought my journal with me, and I read to him the letter I had written him some months before. He was quiet and thoughtful as I read to him my belief that this world is merely one frame in a much larger picture. He watched me as I spoke of my assurance that death is but a journey. Finally, I finished the essay. David did not speak, only nodded and smiled.

"It is just a journey, isn't it?" David asked, his eyes closing, growing heavy under sedation. "I can almost feel that now. It's as if I'm slowly going down a long hill. It's not unpleasant." I knew David was telling the truth. He wasn't in an unpleasant state at all.

"The hard part is over, David." I watched the shallow rising and falling of his chest. His breathing was raspy and rustling—like wind through old, dried leaves.

David was weary and physically spent. Yet he was calm. The Forces that ran this corner of the universe saw to it that David didn't have to agonize to the end. He didn't have to, like many people with AIDS, vomit or convulse or drown in pneumonia. For that, I was grateful. *He's been through enough*, I thought.

Before I began the meditation, he opened his eyes and said, "You've been terrific, Rob. Thanks." I felt an overwhelming sense of gratitude to be a part of David's life, as well as his death. Now, I knew it was time to let him go. During the meditation, I softly spoke of the light that was directly in front of him, surrounding him, comforting him. I told of the spiritual helpers and guides who were there for him, to guide him to the other side.

"You are free to fly," I said at the last. By the time I finished the meditation, David was sound asleep. I sat with him for a time in silence. My mind was reliving the pictures of my months with David. Time existed in a jumbled context in my memories. Had it really only been six months since I'd met David and his family? The events that could be measured in mere days, I knew, would stay with me a lifetime. In silence I reflected over those months and just held David's hand. This was all that was necessary now.

The silence that transcends words. Kübler-Ross was right.

Before I left his room, I turned from the door and looked back at him for the last time. I remembered what Edgar Cayce had said—that "it is not all of life to live, nor yet all of death to die."

Looking at David, much older than his twenty-five years, I realized the hard part was indeed over. In some ways perhaps I envied him. The hard part really *is* the living, not the dying. Day-to-day existence is, at times, a great trial. But now his transition would be a welcome release. The instructor from the training seminar had been right; this had been one of the most brutal, yet one of the most rewarding, experiences of my life.

The reward was nothing tangible. In coming to terms with David's death and dying, I somehow felt I had come to terms with my own. But more, it was an appreciation of how creatively David went on with his life and living. I had a lot to learn there.

"Bye, David," I said quietly at his door. "I love you." As I left the hospital, the evening was alive with the smells of late spring, early summer.

———

I drove back to Morgan and stopped off at Marianne's. It was my birthday, and she gave me a beautiful rose from David's garden in a bronze vase.

"It's the biggest one I could find," she said. "But for some reason there's no scent to it." She held it up for me and, oddly enough, there wasn't a hint of fragrance. I hugged her; laughing, I told her only David could grow roses that size; it took both hands to carry it.

I took the rose home and Mom put it in the living room, awed at the size of it. She then pointed out the spider-plant start that David had given her. It was at home and thriving in the "jungle" in our living room. It was growing faster than any other plant in the house.

"It's just amazing," Mom said, marveling at the spider plant as well as at the rose.

———

The day after my birthday, June 6, 1986, David painlessly left this world. He slipped into a coma, his blood pressure gradually dropped, and he quietly stopped breathing. The hospice center called Marianne when his blood pressure began to drop, but by the time she arrived at the center, David was gone. I received word of his death from the hospice center. Strange, I didn't know whether to grieve or to celebrate—grieve for his passing or celebrate his new life. How do you reconcile the knowing that a soul survives and is alive with the person's absence? Is that why we grieve? I think it is. Not that our friends are dead, but that they are gone from us.

I drove home from work feeling lost, alone, and relieved—an incredible mix of emotions. I missed David, yet I knew he was free. I had prepared for this moment for months, but there really is no preparation for a friend's passing, even when it's expected.

I had a running conversation with David the whole way

home. Perhaps it was my way of dealing with his death, but I remembered from the Cayce readings that it is important to let go of those who have gone on. Cayce said that those who have died are often listening for those still on earth to let them know it's all right to move on, to let go. I kept telling David to go to the light and to put in a good word for me when he got there.

As I drove westward toward Morgan, there was a picturesque sky in front of me—one David surely would have liked.

"It *is* a beautiful sunset," I said aloud. He felt very near.

When I arrived home, my mother met me at the door with a sad, but puzzled expression on her face.

"I'm so sorry, Rob."

I nodded.

"I've got something to show you," she said, walking into the living room. "This morning when I was downstairs, I could have sworn I smelled roses. It was very strong. Then I got the telephone call from Marianne that David had died, and I smelled roses through the whole house!" Mom was holding the bronze vase with the one rose. I could smell it from three feet away.

How appropriate, David, I thought.

"What in the world do you make of this?" Mom asked. "I mean—I *know* there wasn't a fragrance to this rose yesterday."

"I think he's trying to tell us he made it just fine," I said.

The rose—a small token and gift from David through Marianne—forever confirmed my views that death really is but a journey. To this day Mom still talks about the "miraculous" rose from David.

I then understood why David's suicide attempt wasn't successful. For whatever reason he had to go the rest of the distance to the natural end of his life. He had to pass through a very dark night of the soul to reach the dawn. Crucifixion before resurrection. I took the phenomenon of the rose to be an assurance beyond words from David that said, "I'm O.K. All is well." David used the beloved voice of nature to convey his message, the instrument that had been so dear to him while on earth. Not only had his passage illuminated my own life, but it deeply touched my mother's and father's as well.

"David is a very special soul," Mom said. She said, *"David is . . . "* Even she felt the truth that he survived. Her words comforted me.

I drove to meet Marianne at her house. I found her in the back yard, looking at David's flowers.

We hugged each other, and she was smiling through the tears.

"God, but I miss him," Marianne said. Her tears came freely. "I keep asking myself why I had to lose two sons." Trying to choke back my own tears, I told her a passage I had read some years back that was so simple and yet gave me the strength to go on:

One day, you will understand all things. It was from a Cayce reading that helped someone face the hard days of grief.

"Oh, I do hope that's true," Marianne said. "I need to understand . . . so badly." We stood in the yard for some moments, holding onto each other. Finally, when I trusted my voice, I shared with her the story of the scent of the rose. She was happy for it. Like me, Marianne took the experience as an assurance.

"One way or another, David always had to get the last word in," Marianne said, smiling. We stood in the silence, feeling the coming of summer.

"David really is O.K. now, isn't he?" Marianne asked.

I looked at the roses, the spring flowers, the dusk. It was a perfect evening.

"I know he is, Marianne," I said. "I know it with all my heart."

I put my arm around her and we slowly walked to the house. I remembered the passage from *Illusions*: "What the caterpillar calls the end of the world, the Master calls a butterfly."

I hoped that we had helped David to find his wings.

Epilogue

O n a warm April day in 1990, Dr. Martin B. Kleiman, an Indianapolis physician, announced that Ryan White had died after a seven-year battle with AIDS. "He was the boy next door," said Dr. Kleiman, "who first showed to a stunned nation that no one is safe from AIDS. He had no bitterness. With an honest simplicity, his was the voice that many, if not most, first heard—even though his was not the first voice."

Ryan did not die in Kokomo, Indiana.

Even though the White family won their court battle that would allow Ryan to go back to school, the emotional scars of the wounds inflicted by an ignorant community ran deep. It would be simpler to start life anew, in a place they would be welcomed. Ryan and his family moved to the nearby town of Cicero and were welcomed with open arms. Ryan fulfilled his dream and graduated from high school in Cicero, Indiana.

Through a series of what appeared to be personal, medical, and social catastrophic events, Ryan White went on to become the nation's leading spokesperson on AIDS education. Had sectors of Kokomo, Indiana, not ostracized Ryan and his family, not forced them into court nor onto the front pages of the newspapers, I believe that the world would be far less educated than it is today about Acquired Immune Deficiency Syndrome.

"He changed my life," one of Ryan's friends said upon hearing of his death.

"He changed the whole country," said another friend.

Indeed he did. Out of Ryan's pain and suffering, America took note and listened and, I hope, learned.

The night before Ryan's death, Elton John was in Indianapolis performing a concert. He had become a close friend and supporter of the White family and had canceled all other concert engagements to stay with Ryan and his family at the Reilly Children's Hospital. The night of his concert at the Hoosier Dome, Elton John dedicated *Candle in the Wind* to Ryan, who lay comatose in the hospital.

Jeanne White sat in a chair next her dying son that final night. "I knew that somebody had to educate the world about this disease," she said. "I'm just sorry it had to be you, Ryan."

What I once considered unjust and intolerable—specifically the plight of Ryan and his family—became a beacon of light and understanding to an ignorant world. Hard as the lesson is, there is always a sacrifice before wisdom is attained.

After David's death, I went on to be a support person for many people with AIDS and came to know the families as well. David taught me that people sometimes need help in letting go. Edgar Cayce's concept that death is sometimes a healing is part of that letting go. Initially, it was very difficult for me to relinquish the idea that "If I can get them motivated, they will get well and survive." In the cases that I have had, helping patients get well has not been part of my purpose. Because I have faced my fears of death and dying and have come to an understanding—absent of fear—my purpose has been to help people comprehend that death is merely a transition to another realm of consciousness. That is the majority of my work today with the terminally ill.

Medically and scientifically there is still so much that has yet to be discovered about AIDS. For instance, there are more than 6,000 cases of AIDS that have been reported to the Centers for Disease Control in which the patients have no presence of HIV, the virus believed to be the cause of full-blown AIDS. In many ways, we're just *beginning* to understand Acquired Immune Deficiency Syndrome, medically as well as socially.

Today I find myself sometimes frustrated with the public's reluctance to deal head-on with the AIDS epidemic. As much as has been learned about AIDS, ignorance and misinformation remain. People are still being abandoned in certain sectors of society. Some medical people still refuse to touch a person with AIDS; there are still misconceptions and fear. In the city where I am a resident, AIDS education has been removed from mandatory health classes and placed in a "humanities" course that is *optional* for high school students. In other words, AIDS prevention and education is not being taught to all teen-agers. Statistics show that the lack of education is taking its toll: In a recent blood drive at a high school, eight out of eighty students who donated blood tested positive for having the virus associated with AIDS—ten percent of the students. *Teen-agers.* This school is not in a metropolitan area like New York City, San Francisco, or Fort Lauderdale. It is in a medium-sized southern city. These statistics show that today's youth—our future generation—is in trouble.

In the U.S. alone, as of the end of September 1993, there have been 339,250 documented cases of AIDS in the United States.

Of that number, 204,390 have died.

Bibliography/Suggested Reading

Bach, Richard. *Illusions.* New York, N.Y.: Delacorte Press/ Eleanor Friede, 1977.

Baker, M.E. Penny. *Meditation: A Step Beyond with Edgar Cayce,* with foreword by Hugh Lynn Cayce. Garden City, N.Y.: Doubleday, 1973.

Bosnak, Robert. *Dreaming with an AIDS Patient.* Boston, Mass.: Shambhala Publications, Inc., 1989.

Cayce, Hugh Lynn. *Venture Inward.* New York, N.Y.: Harper & Row, 1964.

Dilley, James W.; Helquist, Michael; Pies, Cheri. *Face to Face: A Guide to AIDS Counseling.* San Francisco, Calif.: University of California, AIDS Health Project, 1989.

Foundation, Edgar Cayce. *On Life and Death—The Edgar Cayce Readings, Volume I.* Library Series. Virginia Beach, Va.,

A.R.E. Press, 1973.

Gibran, Kahlil. *Jesus the Son of Man.* New York, N.Y.: Alfred A. Knopf, 1928.

Gill, Derek. *Quest—The Life of Elisabeth Kübler-Ross.* New York, N.Y.: Ballantine Books, 1980.

Kübler-Ross, Elisabeth. *AIDS—The Ultimate Challenge.* New York, N.Y.: Macmillan Publishing, 1987.

Kübler-Ross, Elisabeth. *On Death and Dying.* New York, N.Y.: Macmillan Publishing, 1969.

Moody, Raymond A. *Life After Life.* New York, N.Y.: Bantam/Mockingbird Books, 1975.

Moody, Raymond A. *Reflections on Life After Life.* New York, N.Y.: Bantam/Mockingbird Books, 1977.

Peabody, Barbara. *The Screaming Room.* San Diego, Calif.: Oak Tree Publications, Inc., 1986.

Shilts, Randy. *And the Band Played On: People, Politics, and the AIDS Epidemic.* New York, N.Y.: St. Martin's Press, 1987.

White, Ryan, with Ann Marie Cunningham. *Ryan White: My Own Story.* New York, N.Y.: Dial Books, 1991.

Whitmore, George. *Someone Was Here—Profiles in the AIDS Epidemic.* New York, N.Y.: New American Library, 1988.

About the Author

Robert J. Grant currently lives and works in Virginia Beach, Va., where he is a free-lance writer, publicist, and lecturer. He regularly gives talks, workshops, and seminars dealing with death and dying, creative visualization, near-death experiences, and AIDS.

What Is A.R.E.?

The Association for Research and Enlightenment, Inc. (A.R.E.®), is the international headquarters for the work of Edgar Cayce (1877-1945), who is considered the best-documented psychic of the twentieth century. Founded in 1931, the A.R.E. consists of a community of people from all walks of life and spiritual traditions, who have found meaningful and life-transformative insights from the readings of Edgar Cayce.

Although A.R.E. headquarters is located in Virginia Beach, Virginia—where visitors are always welcome—the A.R.E. community is a global network of individuals who offer conferences, educational activities, and fellowship around the world. People of every age are invited to participate in programs that focus on such topics as holistic health, dreams, reincarnation, ESP, the power of the mind, meditation, and personal spirituality.

In addition to study groups and various activities, the A.R.E. offers membership benefits and services, a bimonthly magazine, a newsletter, extracts from the Cayce readings, conferences, international tours, a massage school curriculum, an impressive volunteer network, a retreat-type camp for children and adults, and A.R.E. contacts around the world. A.R.E. also maintains an affiliation with Atlantic University, which offers a master's degree program in Transpersonal Studies.

For additional information about A.R.E. activities hosted near you, please contact:

A.R.E.
67th St. and Atlantic Ave.
P.O. Box 595
Virginia Beach, VA 23451-0595
(804) 428-3588

A.R.E. Press

A.R.E. Press is a publisher and distributor of books, audiotapes, and videos that offer guidance for a more fulfilling life. Our products are based on, or are compatible with, the concepts in the psychic readings of Edgar Cayce.

We especially seek to create products which carry forward the inspirational story of individuals who have made practical application of the Cayce legacy.

For a free catalog, please write to A.R.E. Press at the address below or call toll free 1-800-723-1112. For any other information, please call 804-428-3588.

> A.R.E. Press
> Sixty-Eighth & Atlantic Avenue
> P.O. Box 656
> Virginia Beach, VA 23451-0656